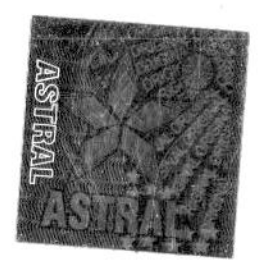

Field cum Laboratory Procedures in Animal Health Care

Field cum Laboratory Procedures in Animal Health Care

by
Zahoor A. Pampori

2003

DAYA PUBLISHING HOUSE
Delhi - 110 035

ISBN 81-7035-314-9

Published by : **Daya Publishing House**
1123/74, Deva Ram Park
Tri Nagar, Delhi - 110 035
Phone : 27103999
Fax : (011) 27199029
e-mail : dayabooks@vsnl.com
website : www.dayabooks.com

Showroom : 4762-63/23, Ansari Road, Darya Ganj,
New Delhi - 110 002
Phone: 23245578, 23244987

Laser Typesetting : **Classic Computer Services**
Delhi - 110 035

Printed at : **Chawla Offset Printers**
Delhi - 110 052

PRINTED IN INDIA

Foreword I

Better human health cannot be dreamed of unless animal care is given due attention. The well being of livestock largely depends on better management, early detection of ailment and its effective treatment and control. Even if our livestock population contributes significantly towards the economic development, yet due attention is not being given for their upkeep. In our state farmers have not yet tasted the fruits of available modem techniques/facilities in animal health care. This is probably because of lack of awareness among public as also poor feed back from the field besides lack of expertise in the veterinary field staff. It is perhaps, this subtle feeling and the inspiration of staff of the Institute of Animal Health, Zakura, Srinagar that has made the author, who has been working in the institute, to write the book which contains valuable information about collection, preservation and transportation of test materials, besides a worthy comprehensive table, for arriving at early and definite diagnosis of a disease.

I personally feel delighted to see one of my associates venturing this task and am confident that this book would be helpful to the field veterinary staff as also the laboratory personnel.

(Dr. N.A. Khan)
Joint Director,
Institute of Animal Health, Zakura

Foreword II

It is a matter of immense pleasure to have in my hands the manuscript of the book "Field cum Laboratory Procedures in Animal Health Care". The book, a timely and laudable effort by our young veterinary scientist Dr. Z.A. Pampori should serve as a very useful guide to the field and laboratory workers alike.

It is often seen that excellent advanced research/diagnostic facilities cannot realize their full potential because of insufficient, unrelated, or unscrupulously collected, preserved and transported test materials. One of the other factors influencing the ultimate results obtained could be a flaw in the technique employed in the laboratory. This book is an attempt to preclude such possibilities.

I am confident that this book can be used as a guide manual by field veterinarians, paravets, farm owners and managers, diagnostic laboratories and other institutions related to the field of livestock industry and research work.

I congratulate the author for his creative venture and expect him to continue his creative efforts further.

(Dr.M.M.Ahmad)
Director,
Animal Husbandry Department,
Kashmir, J&K State

From Dean's Desk

In a rapidly developing field of scientific endeavour, technical approaches that are of paramount importance for progress in the field are not static but under go constant change. The impact of new technology associated with these developments has been to create hopes for the diagnosis and control of numerous disorders of livestock including poultry. The careful evaluation of the history and occurrence of multifactorial disease in the laboratory will facilitate appropriate corrective measures. Dr. Z.A. Pampori has done a commendable job in structuring and editing this volume of handbook of *Field cum Laboratory Procedures in Animal Health Care.* The handbook/laboratory manual, has comprehensive coverage on collection, preservation, transportation and processing of the samples/suspected material in the laboratory for disease diagnosis. The author has elucidated the suitable methodologies for washing, sterilization of laboratory wares, collection of material for laboratory diagnosis, handling of suspected material in the laboratory, isolation and identification of bacteria, fungi, viruses and parasites.

The author has included separate chapters on care and management of laboratory animals, production of common livestock and poultry vaccines, physiological profile of different animals, tabular representation of animal diseases, their diagnosis and the trace chart containing valuable information is an added feature of this book.

I am sure that this handbook will be of immense value and beneficial to the students, veterinarians and paravets in the disease investigation laboratories, in the biological institutes and in the field.

DR. A.S. BUCHH

Dean/Professor and Head
Division of Microbiology & Immunology,
Faculty of Veterinary Sciences and A.H.,
SKUAST, Kashmir

Preface

A globally significant role for the Indian livestock system depends critically on India's ability to control and eradicate the animal diseases. Though the livestock sector contributes an estimated 8.4% to the country GDP and 35.85% of the agricultural out put, yet livestock diseases are the most important constraints to profitable animal production. Acute infectious diseases on one hand decrease the animal population and chronic diseases on the other hand results in production losses. India contributes about 19% of the world cattle and buffalo population and 20% that of goats besides appreciable proportion of sheep and poultry. India has become highest milk producer in the world. Kashmir division has livestock population of 38 lakh and milk production 290 lakh tons, making 290ml milk available per person per day. Present animal disease scenario has increased the importance and responsibility of a veterinarian in field as well as in laboratory, while demanding reliable and quick disease diagnosis, besides treatment. There are, no doubt, reliable and quick diagnostic tools available in the country but disease diagnosis, while employing them, cannot be achieved from any laboratory unless the relevant and desirable sample is collected, handled, preserved and transported to the diagnostic centre in the best possible manner. It becomes necessary for a veterinarian to know what materials are required to be collected for disease diagnosis and similarly laboratory persons must be aware of the tests/techniques to be employed for an early diagnosis of a disease. Realizing the need and responsibility, this book has been designed to impart the basic knowledge of collection, preservation, transportation of samples required for diagnosis of a disease besides providing preliminary information about the techniques / tests/ procedures employed in the field and laboratory. An attempt has been made to frame a trace chart of practical guidelines to be followed in the diagnosis of a particular disease. This book also includes physiological profile of various parameters in domestic animals besides tips for better care and management of laboratory animals. I hope this book shall prove valuable for the field veterinarians, laboratories and veterinary students.

In the foremost I offer my heartfelt devotions to Almighty. Help, inspiration and encouragement rendered by Dr. M. M. Ahmad (Director,Animal Husbandry,Kashmir), Dr. N.K. Kuda (Ex.Director), Dr. A. Khan (Joint Director), Dr. A.M. Qureshi (Dy.Director), Dr. Saleem Iqbal (HOD, Vety. Physiology, FVSc.), Dr. A.K. Bhat, Dr. J.L. Matoo, Dr. V.K. Koul, Dr. A.K. Raina, Dr. M. Chesti, Dr. M. Naqati, Dr. F.A. Jan, Dr. K.A. Shah, Dr. M. Shaheen, Dr. M. Saleem, Dr. Neelofer, Dr. Shaista, Mushtaq A. Shah,G.A.Fazli, M.Shafi and M. Ashraf is gratefully acknowledged. I tender my deep sense of regards, love and affection to my parents and dependents for their encouragement and forbearance during my undertaking this piece of work.

In undertaking this task, errors and omissions are inescapable and I welcome your corrections, comments and suggestions.

Zahoor A. Pampori

Contents

Chapter 1
Washing and Sterilization of Laboratory Wares

1.1. WASHING

For any laboratory procedure, it is necessary that all kinds of laboratory wares should be clean, dirt, dust and grease free. For microbiological use, laboratory wares must be free from microbes also.

Laboratory wares should be cleaned by a cleansing agent that removes all traces of dirt or dust with no residual precipitation of cleansing agent. Do not use soap. A detergent should be used to clean the wares. Detergent to be used should have qualities like;

1. It should not contain free alkali,
2. It should soften water,
3. It should be quickly and completely soluble in water,
4. It should not precipitate,
5. It should lower the surface tension and easily be rinsed,
6. It should have good wetting quality besides being non-irritant.

The laboratory wares should be soaked for a short time in wash tubs with 1% detergent warm water. Scrubbing of the wares should be done wherever necessary with a brush. The wares should be then rinsed with running warm water or better distilled or deionized water for at least three times. It is advisable to rinse the wares with distil water when in use for microbiology. Washed wares are set on a clean dry surface to drain and dry.

The laboratory wares with agar, jelly or paraffin should be first autoclaved or submerged in large container and then heated to boil. Thereafter, washing is followed as discussed. However, in advanced laboratories there are mechanical washers used for washing different types of laboratory wares.

The used microscopic slides with immersion oil should be first washed with xylol, rinsed with tap water and then immersed in 1:1000 solution of nitric acid for over night, then rinsed thoroughly and dried with tissue paper. New slides should be washed with water and placed in 95% alcohol for 15 minutes and then dried with tissue paper.

After washing and drying, the laboratory wares to be sterilized should be wrapped with brown paper and mouths plugged with cotton plug or corks to ensure maintenance of sterility.

1.2. STERILIZATION

Sterilization is a process of destroying germs including spores. Sterilization can be effected in a variety of ways depending upon the nature of material to be sterilized like instruments, laboratory wares, equipments, drugs or culture media etc. The sterilization methods are discussed hereunder.

1.2.a. Heat Sterilization

Heat can be applied for sterilization in two forms, the dry heat and the moist heat.

Sterilization by Dry Heat

Sterilization is effected at a temperature of 160 °C for 1 hour or 180°C for 30 minutes that is sufficient to kill most of the resistant spores. Dry heat is believed to kill the organisms by destructive oxidation of essential cell constituents. This type of sterilization is employed for glass wares, metallic wares or other goods which are not spoiled by high temperature and anhydrous fats, oils and powders which are impermeable to moisture.

Inoculating wires, loops, points of forceps are sterilized by keeping them in a burner flame until red hot. Scalpels, needles, mouths of culture tubes, cotton plugs or glass slides are sterilized by passing them through the burner flame with out making them red hot.

Most of the glass wares used in the laboratory are sterilized in electric hot air ovens maintained at a constant temperature of 160°C or 180°C.

Infra red radiation is a new method of dry heat sterilization. In this method infra red rays from an electrically heated element are directed to an object to be sterilized and a temperature of 180°C is attained. This method is being employed in sterilization of surgical instruments.

Sterilization by Moist Heat

It requires moist heat at 121°C for 15 to 30 minutes to kill most resistant spores. Moist heat is believed to kill organisms by coagulating and denaturing their enzymes and structural proteins. All culture media, liquids, rubber and plastic wares are sterilized by moist heat treatment which can be best achieved through saturated steam under increased pressure.

Pasteurization

Sterilization by moist heat can be achieved at temperatures below 100°C and where temperature is raised to 63°C for 30 minutes or 72°C for 20 seconds, it is referred as pasteurization. This kind of sterilization is some times employed in body fluids or serum which contains coagulable proteins.

Vaccines from non-sporing bacteria can be sterilized in a vaccine bath maintained at a temperature of 60°c for 1 hour. Moist heat sterilization at 100°C temperature can be achieved by *boiling for 5 to 10 minutes*, sufficient to kill all non-sporing organisms. Although it does not ensure complete sterilization yet has been found satisfactory method of sterilization in conditions where other better methods of sterilization are not available or absolute sterilization is not needed. Various glass wares, instruments and articles can be sterilized by this method and while removing the articles from the boiling water always use sterile forceps for holding them till they dry.

Tyndallization

Exposing the material, to be sterilized, to steam at 100°C for 20 to 45 minutes on each of three successive days is sufficient to kill the vegetative organisms and the process is called tyndallization. This method of sterilization is generally used in sterilizing media with sugars which otherwise get decomposed on higher temperatures or gelatin which fails to solidify after prolonged heating.

Autoclaving

Sterilization by moist heat is best achieved in autoclave, which is the most reliable method of sterilization and widely used for sterilization of culture media and surgical tools. It is conveniently employed for sterilization of plastic or rubber wares, corks or stoppers that do with- stand autoclaving. The principle that works in autoclave is that water is boiled within a closed vessel at increased pressure and the temperature at which it boils or temperature of steam it forms rises above 100°C. This way autoclave provides moist heat at temperature higher than 100°C. Hot saturated steam effects sterilization by virtue of its high temperature, condensation of steam into small volume of water, on contact with cooler surface, and contraction of volume invites more steam to the site and the process continues until material is heated to the temperature of steam which ensures the killing of microbes. Once material has obtained the temperature of steam, the holding temperature is minimum (12 to 20 minute at not less than 121°Cor 15 lbs per sq.inch gauge pressure or 30 to 45 minutes at not less than 115°C or 10 lbs per sq.inch gauge pressure).

1.2.b. Sterilization by Radiation

Ultra Violet Radiation

It is one of the methods of sterilization involving the rays of wave length of 330mu or below. The shortest ultraviolet rays in sun light that reach the earth are having wave length of 290 mu. Radiation of 240 –280 mu can be produced by mercury vapour lamps, ultra violet rods. Ultra violet rays from suitably shielded lamps have been used to reduce the number of bacteria in the atmosphere, hence employed in sterilization of operation theaters, laboratories, working hoods (laminar flow) etc.

Ionizing Radiation

It is a method of sterilization that involves high speed electrons, X- *rays and Gamma rays* that are obtained from a machine or isotope such as cobalt 60. This type of sterilization is commercially worth in sterilizing large amounts of pre-packed disposable items such as plastic syringes or catheters which do not with stand heat. It is much more powerful than ultra violet radiation.

1.2.c. Sterilization by Filtration

This method of sterilization involves use of special filters through which material to be sterilized is allowed to pass. This method is especially useful in preparation of soluble products of bacterial growth such as toxins and in sterilization of culture media, liquids that are heat labile such as serum and antibiotic solutions. Sterilization is effected by the use of filters having pores smaller than the microbes which are thus arrested. Filters with pore diameter of 0.75µ or less are able to retain bacteria and filters are also now available with pore diameter less enough to arrest the viruses.

There are many types of filters like, Berkefield filters, Chamberland filters, Seitz filters, Sintered glass filters or Membrane filters. Membrane filters are sterilized itself by steaming where as others by autoclaving.

1.2.d. Sterilization by Chemical Agents

Though absolute sterilization is not achieved by using agents widely grouped as antiseptics and disinfectants yet these are of paramount importance in decontaminating the surfaces.

Antiseptics are non toxic chemical agents, able to kill or restrict the growth of micro-organisms, used tropically in animate things.

Disinfectants are more potent but toxic agents, able to destroy the micro-organisms, suited for application in inanimate objects.

Chloroform is sometimes used in sterilization and preservation of serum at 0.25% and can be removed by heating at 56°C.

Phenol, cresol and Lysol are powerful antiseptics, which are used in sterilizing surgical instruments and discarded cultures. Lysol is used in 3% solution, where as phenol 0.5% and cresol 0.1% for preservation of serum and vaccines.

Quaternary ammonium compounds such as Benzalkonium chloride are surface active compounds which are highly bactericidal. Alcohol and iodophores are conveniently used to reduce and eliminate the superficial flora from the skin surfaces. Alcohol causes the denaturation of proteins and rapidly kills vegetative bacteria, when used as 70-90% aqueous solution. Commonly used alcohols are isopropyl alcohol (90-95%) or ethanol (70-90%). Iodine is an effective chemical agent that acts by oxidizing essential components of the microbial cell. It is commonly used as tincture of 2% iodine in 50% alcohol.

Mercuric chloride is used sometimes as a disinfectant in 1:1000 dilutions or Merthiolate in 1:10000 dilutions for preservation of antitoxin and other sera.

Formalin is used to kill and fix the bacterial cultures and suspensions at 0.5 to 1% in solution.

Chlorine is a very effective oxidizing lethal agent for microbes. Chlorine in concentration less than 1ppm kills most of vegetative bacteria and viruses when used in decontamination of water.

1.2.e. Sterilization by Gases

Heat labile goods or appliances can conveniently be sterilized by exposing to ethylene oxide gas or formaldehyde gas.

Formaldehyde gas is used to sterilize the articles that are not completely wetted with solution or damaged by wetting. Articles like shoes, brushes, incubating chambers and even rooms are disinfected by formaldehyde gas when the chambers are made leak-proof. 50ml formalin with 1000ml water is boiled per 100cu.feet of air space and maintained for 4 to 24 hours. Ammonia solution is introduced to neutralize the formaldehyde.

Ethylene oxide is also a highly lethal gaseous sterilizer that kills bacteria, viruses and even spores. It is used in the sterilization of heat labile articles like plastic and rubber wares, blankets, pharmaceutical products or complex apparatuses.10%ethylene oxide in carbon dioxide or in halogenated hydrocarbons can be employed for sterilization.

Chapter 2

General Recommendations in Handling Samples for Laboratory Diagnosis

The animal disease diagnosis, while employing different diagnostic techniques or procedures, can not be achieved from any laboratory unless the correct sample is acquired, handled, preserved in the best possible manner and transported to the laboratory for processing before it is deteriorated. No reliance can be placed on the results obtained by different laboratory tests from poor, inadequate or badly preserved samples. It is very important for a veterinarian to know exactly what materials or samples are required by the laboratory before collecting any sample for the diagnosis of a disease.

2.1. General Recommendations for Sample Collection and Transportation

1. Sample must be as fresh as possible, obtained and preserved in right manner.
2. Sample must be properly labeled and easily identifiable.
3. Sample must carry information like owner's name and address, species, age, clinical signs or necropsy findings, tentative diagnosis and type of sample submitted.
4. Sample must bear information about exact estimation or any specific test to be employed.
5. Sample must be transported to the laboratory as early as possible in air tight, clean or sterilized glass or plastic containers.

6. Containers containing sample must be packed properly to avoid any breakage or leakage during transit.

The samples thus collected need to be transported to the laboratory in an atmosphere that maintains the quality of sample for laboratory diagnosis. Where the samples are required to be transported under refrigeration temperature (4-10°C) or frozen state, the following procedure can be conveniently followed;

a. Place the sample container in a water proof insulated container, containing ice, that will keep the sample cool for 12 to 20 hours.

b. Sample, if transported personally, can be held in a thermosflask with ice.

c. Put the sample in the plastic bag and surround it with dry ice (solid carbon dioxide) in an air proof box.

2.2. General Recommendations for Sample Selection

Samples, for laboratory diagnosis of a disease, can be taken either from live animals or from dead after postmortem and the samples so collected are subjected to different laboratory tests. Depending upon the investigations or tests, to be employed, certain precautions are needed to be taken at the time of sample collection. These can be conveniently grouped as under;

2.2.a. Samples for Bacteriological Evaluation

The samples for culture and isolation of organisms must be taken while observing strict aseptic measures to exclude any contamination from surrounding areas or tissues or atmosphere. The operator should ensure that while collecting sample he is not transporting contamination from his hands, clothes or exhalation for which sterile gloves, apron and masks are used. The areas from which samples are to be taken should be thoroughly cleaned with antiseptic like alcohol, sprit or betadine. The samples should be collected in sterilized containers and transported under refrigeration temperature. The body fluids like blood, peritoneal fluid, cerebrospinal fluid, synovial fluid can be aspirated using sterile disposable syringes and transported as such in the syringe devoid of any air in the syringe. When the samples are taken through a contaminated area like uterine swabs, use of special enclosed cervical swabs is recommended, while using disposable sterile gloves.

Swabs are of value in many instances for the transport of infectious material to the lab. Where there is apprehension of desiccation during transportation, it is advisable to place the swabs in sterile non-nutritional transport medium. Sterilized disposable swabs are available commercially for the said purpose. Swabs can also be prepared by attaching absorbent cotton to the end of a thin stick or a wire with a rubber band or thread, wrapped in a paper and then autoclaved.

Transtracheal aspiration and bronchial brush are useful for collecting material for culture.

Live, acutely sick animals that can be sacrificed and necropsied are usually the best source of specimens. Samples at necropsy should contain the obvious lesions, if present and if not, samples (about ½ ounce or 1x2 in.) should be submitted from liver, kidneys, spleen, intestine and lymphnodes. The samples should be taken at the margins of diseased and normal tissue. Intestines should be ligated at the cut ends and packed separately. Specimens can conveniently be shipped in thermocool boxes containing sufficient amount of ice. However, where delay is inevitable, dry ice with plenty of insulation is preferred.

Cauterization of the surface with red hot spatula, before taking samples from deeper areas or from necropsy material, also helps reduce contamination. Never use histological fixatives or unsterile additives if at all to be added

Special commercial transport systems are available for transporting the materials suspected of containing anaerobs.

2.2.b. Samples for Viral and Mycoplasma Isolation

For isolation of viruses and mycoplasma from the collected samples, it is obligatory to transport the material in transport medium. Samples should be held in refrigeration temperature but should not freeze. Tissues from the lesions or at necropsy should not be less than2g (2-5 g) and placed in 10 times of its volume of transport medium or tissue culture medium.

Viral transport medium is basically consisting of Hank's solution with a protein (1% albumin), a buffer and antibiotics (penicillin and streptomycin and or polymixin B). 50% glycerin phosphate buffer saline (one part of glycerin + one part of phosphate buffer saline) is widely used. Very common substitute for the transport medium is boiled skimmed milk. Fresh fecal samples can be used with out transport medium for identification of enteric viruses.

Mycoplasma transport medium is basically Brain- heart infusion broth, yeast extract, antifungal (nystatin) and antibiotics (ampicillin).

In viral infection, it is recommended that paired serum samples, one at the onset of disease and other 2-3 weeks after the first sample, should be submitted for confirmation of the disease. The appreciable increase in the antibody titer between acute and convalescent sera is a significant indicator of viral infection.

Serum should be shipped in deep frozen state or on dry ice where as blood preferably in wet ice or with coolant but not frozen. Unclotted whole blood can be conveniently submitted in 5 ml amount in EDTA.

2.2.c. Samples for Mycological Evaluation

The majority of diseases caused by pathogenic fungi or yeast are those which produce superficial lesions of skin and mucous membranes like Microsporum, Trichophyton or Epidermophyton. The diseases like pulmonary or intestinal actinomycosis, aspergillosis, systemic histoplas-mosis or cryptococosis are clinically less recognized, with out any initial local lesions and are diagnosed very late or only at autopsy. Specimens should be taken from all lesions preferably from the edges with sterile instruments and collected in sterile containers. Skin scrapings should be taken after cleansing the area with 70% alcohol. Material should be dispatched to the laboratory with out any delay as the materials more than 3-4 hours old are less apt to prove satisfactory. In case of pustule or abscess like lesions, it is advisable to aspirate the material with the help of sterilized syringes avoiding opening of the lesions. In suspected lung mycosis sputum or a fragment of tissue obtained bronchoscopically should be collected and examined. Material collected for mycological evaluation should be divided into three parts, one for direct microscopic examination, second for culture and third for animal inoculation and other special tests. Direct examination of samples in many instances is sufficient for diagnosis of fungus but for establishing the identity of species it is necessary to adopt other methods like culture etc.

2.2.d. Samples for Toxicological Evaluation

For toxicological investigation veterinarian must be quite clear as to what material will yield the results and should clearly mention the estimations required. It is of great value to submit the suspected source of the toxicity when ever possible. About 500ml of Ruminal, abomasal or stomach contents, besides liver (50g atleast), vomitus, perirenal fat, heparinized blood (10ml), faeces (5-10g) and urine(60ml), are collected and sent to the laboratory. When plant or food poisoning is suspected, the stem, leaves, flowers, fruits, stored grains, feed or hay should be collected and dispatched to the forensic laboratory in closed sealed containers under refrigeration temperature to avoid growth of bacteria and fungi. Sections of the tissue showing gross changes, besides liver and kidney, should be fixed in formalin and sent to the laboratory.

2.2.e. Samples for Biochemical Estimation

The majority of biochemical estimations are carried in serum although plasma can also be used and in that case heparin (1mg per 5 ml blood) is used as anticoagulant. The estimations should be performed as rapidly as possible or the sample should be deep frozen if delay is inevitable. For glucose estimation the fluoride containing anticoagulant should be used. Test kits are commercially available for most of the biochemical estimations.

2.2.f. Samples/Specimens for Histopathology

The materials/specimens for histopathological examination should be collected immediately after death. The material should be taken from the portion representing characteristic lesion preferably from the boundary zone between normal and abnormal tissue and fixed as soon as possible. Slices of tissues, not more than 5mm thick or ½ x 1/5 sq. inch., should be taken. Tissue should not be crushed or tired while collecting.

The most common fixative used for tissue fixation is 10% formal saline (100ml formaldehyde + 900 ml distilled water + 8.5 g sodium chloride) and is well suited for micro anatomical studies of the specimens. Flemming's fluid (Chromic acid 15ml + 4 ml of 2% osmic acid + glacial acetic acid 1ml) or Carony's fluid (absolute alcohol 60ml +chloroform 30ml + glacial acetic acid 10ml) can be used as a fixative for cytological examination. The fixative should be ten to twenty times more than the volume of the tissue and should never be frozen.

The material should be placed in a wide mouth glass container. A cotton pad can be placed below and above the tissue while in formal saline. Label showing the particulars of the specimen, written with a hard black lead pencil, should be placed in side the container and the container itself should also be labeled. The mouth of the container should be well sealed, packed and then dispatched to the concerned lab.

2.2.g. Samples for Parasitological Examinations

Collect fecal samples from the rectum and submit the samples separately in impervious plastic or glass containers in a way to exclude as much air as possible from the container. Samples should be held in refrigeration temperature.

For diagnosis of abomasal worms, serum is submitted for serum pepsinogen determination. For identification of trematodes or nematodes or cestodes, they are preserved in 5% formalin.

Diagnosis of blood parasites requires submission of blood sample in EDTA and or blood smears.

Skin scrapings, hair or wool, should be submitted in a sterile, clean, dry container. Ectoparasites, larvae or snails should be dispatched in a jar with moist cotton or blotting paper to avoid desiccation.

Commercially Available Transport Media

Some of the commercially available transport media, marketed by HIMEDIA, are enlisted here.

1. Buffered glycerol saline base (for transportation and collection of faecal samples).
2. Cary-Blair Medium base (for collection and shipment of clinical samples).
3. Amies transport medium with charcoal (transportation and preservation of microbiological specimens).
4. Specimen preservative medium (for collection, transportation and preservation of stool specimens or rectal swabs for isolation of entero-bacteriaceae).

Chapter 3

Standard Procedures Involved in Collection and Transportation of Samples

3.1. Blood Samples

Blood is a very important sampling material, either clotted or un-clotted, for diagnosis of most of the diseases. The blood can be collected from different animals quite conveniently by adopting the right procedure. It is important to prepare the site of blood collection by shaving or clipping the hair especially in long haired animals and application of alcohol at the site. The syringes and needles used in collection should be sterile, preferably disposable type or self-filling tubes.

Coagulation of blood can be prevented by employing different anticoagulants, the important ones are;

1. *Ethylenediaminetetra acetic acid (EDTA)* can be used at 1 – 2mg per ml of blood.
2. *Heparin* can be used at 0.1 – 0.2mg per ml of blood. Moistening of syringe with 1% heparin solution is sufficient to prevent coagulation of the blood drawn in it.
3. *Sodium citrate* is a commonly used anticoagulant at 1-2mg or 0.1ml of 3.8% solution per ml of blood.
4. *Potassium oxalate or Sodium oxalate* can be used at 2mg per ml of blood.
5. *Sodium fluoride* is preferably used in samples for glucose estimation at 5-10mg per ml of blood.
6. *Acid citrate dextrose(ACD)* is used in preventing coagulation

of blood for transfusion at 25ml per 100ml of blood. It can be prepared by dissolving dextrose-14.7gm, Trisodium citrate-13.2gm, citric acid anhydrous- 4.4gm, in 1 lit. distilled water which can then be sterilized by autoclaving.

In cattle, sheep and horse the blood in good quantity can be collected from *jugular vein*. The vein is raised by putting pressure with the left hand at the base of neck and distended vein can easily be felt. A sterile stout needle of 18 gauge is inserted quickly into the distended vein in upward and inward direction. When the needle is in the vein a jet of blood comes out and can be collected either in a syringe fitted to the needle or in a flask connected to the needle with rubber tubing. After blood is collected, needle is withdrawn quickly and pressure is applied to the puncture wound with a cotton swab to arrest the bleeding. Same vein can be used conveniently for repeated collections.

In cattle *coccygeal vein* at the base of tail is a feasible site of blood collection. The tail is raised and a needle is inserted directly in the mid line at second or third coccygeal intervertebral space. This technique, however, works best with vacutainers. *Mammary vein* can also be used for blood collection in cattle, which appears at the anterior boarder of mammary gland lateral to linea alba.

Pigs can be bled from *ear vein* which is raised by means of a rubber band applied round the base of ear. *Anterior venacava* is a good site for collection of blood in pigs provided the means for restraining the animal are adequate. The carniform cartilage of the sternum is located and a line is drawn from there to the base of the ear. Needle is inserted in this line just anterior to and to one side of the carniform cartilage at an angle of 60 degree. A needle (3.5 cm of 20 gauge) fitted to a syringe with negative pressure is inserted in a posterior direction until blood appears in the syringe.

In dogs and cats blood can be collected from *cephalic or recurrent tarsal veins*, raised by using digital pressure. *Jugular vein* is a good sampling site in debilitated dogs and cats. Cephalic vein can be raised just above carpal joint by applying pressure on the dorsal aspect of the forelimb at the level of elbow. A *marginal ear vein* on the dorsal side of ear can be used conveniently in dogs, cats and other laboratory animals. *Femoral* or *saphenous* vein on medial aspect of the leg between knee and abdomen can also be punctured for blood collection.

In fowl a small amount of blood can be drawn by clipping a small piece of one of the points of comb. However, blood can be collected from a *humeral (wing vein) vein* by holding the bird on its side with breast towards operator and turning the top wing back. Humeral vein is located in the loose fascia on the inner side of the wing. Blood is drawn in a syringe with a 21 to 23 gauge needle fitted to it from the humeral vein.

In rabbit blood can be obtained from *ear veins*. Rub the ear with xylol and alcohol after vigorously filliping the ear with hand. Puncture a marginal vein with large needle and the blood trickles down in drops that can be collected in tubes up to 2-3 ml. Bleeding can be checked by applying pressure to the wound. Blood can be collected directly from the *heart* by thrusting 19 gauge needle, fitted to a syringe, at the point of maximum pulsation on the left side of the chest after strictly disinfecting the site of puncture. 10 to 20 ml of blood can be collected from a 2 kg rabbit at intervals of 2 to 3 weeks.

Guinea pigs can be bled by exposing the large *vessels of neck* by longitudinal incision on one side, after the animal is anesthetized with ether. Vessels are severed and blood collected in tubes by using a funnel but care is taken not to severe the esophagus or trachea. Blood can be aspirated from the *heart* directly, after the animal is held firmly or fastened to a board and lightly anesthetized, by inserting a needle of 21gauge fitted to a syringe at the point of maximum pulsation on the left side of chest. When the needle is in the heart, blood is drawn in the syringe and an amount of 5-15 ml can be aspirated from the heart.

In mice small amount of blood can be collected by *clipping the tail*. However, collection of 1 ml blood requires puncturing of *retro-orbital plexus* of veins by displacing the globe of eye forwards to expose the plexus. Blood can be collected by severing of *great vessels in the axilla*, after skin over thorax and abdomen is reflected under deep anesthesia.

Blood smears can be made by taking a drop of blood or by touching a large drop of blood at one end of a clean, grease free slide. Spread the blood with a second slide with smooth edges, held at an angle of 45 degrees with the under slide by touching the drop of blood. As soon as blood has spread entirely across the end of the spreader slide, with a rather quick movement, push the spreader slide *(do not pull)* towards the other end of the under slide in longitudinal axis. A film neither too thin nor too thick is made and air dried. The smears are then fixed in absolute methyle alcohol for 2 minutes and then air dried.

De-fibrination of blood can be achieved by using sterilized glass beads in a collection flask and gently shaking the blood and beads for a while which arrests the coagulation of blood. It can be either immediately used or held in refrigeration temperature.

For culture, blood on sterile swabs is preferred and transportation under refrigeration in thermos-flask with wet ice or coolant packs is recommended.

Blood for *hematology* should be placed in clean vials with an anticoagulant and mixed gently but thoroughly to prevent coagulation. 5 ml of blood is sufficient for hematology. Blood should be held in refrigeration temperature.

3.2. Serum and Plasma Samples

Blood samples when collected for separation of serum or plasma should be collected carefully avoiding rupture of red cells. Use of wet syringes should be avoided and after aspiration, blood from syringe should be transferred in vials only when needle is removed.

Plasma can be obtained by centrifuging the uncoagulated blood in centrifuge tubes at 3000rpm for ten minutes when the red cells form the pellet at the bottom of the tube and clear fluid, plasma, at the top can be collected carefully by pipetting out, while avoiding red cells.

Serum is collected by drawing the blood in sterilized wide mouth tubes or trays. Blood is allowed to coagulate at room temperature and when clot retracts, it is centrifuged and a straw coloured fluid, the serum, is pipetted out in sterile vials. The serum may also be collected by allowing the blood to coagulate at room temperature and then allowed to stand in refrigeration temperature for overnight, the straw coloured fluid can conveniently be pipetted out as serum.

Serum should be held and transported in clean, sterilized vials preferably in deep frozen state. 2 ml of serum is sufficient for most of the serology for which atleast 5 ml of blood is collected. For long term storage sodium azide @ 0.5% should be added.

It is recommended to send paired samples one at onset of the disease and another two to three weeks later so that recent infection is confirmed by determining the rising antibody titer. Serological tests are generally used as confirmatory tests.

3.3. Urine Samples

Urine samples should be collected either during *micturation* or *at catheterization* taking strict aseptic measures. *Mid flow urine* samples give most reliable results.

For culture purposes the sample should be collected aseptically in sterile and sealed bottles and held in refrigeration temperature. Sample should be subjected to required investigations as immediately as possible and should be transported in refrigeration temperature using wet ice or coolant packs. If leptospira is suspected, 10% formalin should be added to the urine sample at the rate of 7.5%, as the leptospira disintegrates shortly after collection, if not fixed.

3.4. Sputum

It should be collected directly from the animal using sterilized swabs or a spatula and placed in sterile glass or plastic containers to prevent drying of the sample. No preservative is added.

3.5. Serous Cavity Fluids

Samples taken from *pleural or peritoneal cavities* are generally used for bacteriological or cytological studies. Strict aseptic measures should be observed while taking sample. The puncture site is shaved and desensitized with local anesthetics. Chest puncture is performed between *6th and 8th intercostals space* in the lower third of the chest. 3mm dia. sterile needles can be used in large animals and 1mm dia. for small animals. Fluid collected aseptically should be placed in sterile, screw stopper containers with out adding any preservative. However in inflammatory conditions when high protein content is expected in the sample an anticoagulant EDTA (2mg/ml) should be added to prevent coagulation. The sample should be transported under refrigeration temperature.

3.6. Cerebro-spinal Fluid

It can be collected from *cisterna magna* by means of sub-occipital approach or from *spinal sub-arachnoid space* in the lumber region. In all cases the site of puncture is shaved, swabbed with alcohol or sprit and strict asepsis is maintained. Sterile spinal needles are used (3mm x 12 cm in cattle and 1mm x 6cm in dog) for collection only under local anesthetics or sedation or general anesthesia.

In cattle lumber approach is preferred. The needle is inserted in the mid line at the soft depression between the dorsal process of lumber vertebrae and the anterior end of the median sacral crest.

In horse sub-occipital puncture is best. Under general anesthesia, head is flexed vertically until the angle between head and neck is 90^0. Needle is inserted at a point, with the anterior edge of the wings of atlas, in the midline of the neck.

In dogs and cats sub-occipital puncture is a method of choice where as *in sheep and goat* both approaches are satisfactory. The sample should be collected in sterilized, sealed vials and held under refrigeration temperature. No preservative is added. It should be transported to the laboratory immediately and estimations carried out as quickly as possible.

3.7. Synovial Fluid

The puncture site and quantity of fluid will depend upon the type of joint affected. The site of puncture should be shaved, cleaned with absolute alcohol or spirit and strict asepsis observed. The skin and joint capsule is infiltrated with local anesthetics. Short, sterile needles of 18 gauge are used for collection of fluid fitted to a sterile syringe. Fluid should be aspirated and collected in sterile screw stopper containers using anticoagulant EDTA (2mg/ml) or 3.8% sodium citrate(0.1ml/ml). 2-3 ml fluid is sufficient for full range of investigations.

3.8. Milk Samples

Milk is collected directly into clean, sterilized, screw caped, water tight containers. It is advisable to discard first few streaks of milk (milk in teat cistern) before collection and udder should be washed thoroughly and swabbed with alcohol prior to sampling. It should be transported under refrigeration temperature to the laboratory. For milk ring test, avoid colostrum or milk from a cow suffering from mastitis. For milk ELISA tests, milk can be stored in frozen state and a drop of formalin added to it. 25 ml of milk is sufficient for all type investigations.

3.9. Fecal Samples

Fecal samples should be collected directly from the rectum or from the freshly passed feces at floor avoiding straw, soil or any extraneous material. Material is collected in clean, sterile and stoppered containers. Rectal swabs are available for collecting fecal material for culture purpose. For parasitic egg counting the container is tightly filled with material to exclude any air and tightly stoppered before dispatch. Where a delay in processing and examination of faecal samples is unavoidable, they can be preserved by using preservatives like formalin solution, Schaudinn's solution, Polyvinyl alcohol containing Schaudinn's solution and Merthiolate-iodine-formaldehyde (MIF). Specimens and the preservatives must be adequately mixed and one part of faeces is mixed with 7 to 14 parts of preservative. For quantitative analysis like egg count, it is important to standardize the quantity of faeces put into preservative. Formalin preserved specimens are good for survey of helminth infections and MIF for preserving protozoa. Adult worm identification is facilitated by submitting the material in 5% formal-saline.

3.10. Skin Scrapings and Hair Samples

These samples are required for the diagnosis of mite infestation or fungal infection. Skin scrapings are obtained by scraping the skin with the edge of sharp scalpel blade until bleeding. Scrapings should be made from active lesions and several sites should be used. All debris collected should be transferred to a clean dry container and dispatched with out any preservation. Hair samples are used primarily for identification of fungal infections. Samples are best taken from the outer edges of active lesions. Hairs must be pulled out, not cut, and dispatched in sealed clean containers or wrapped in clean paper.

3.11. Biopsy Samples

Bone Marrow Biopsy

It can be satisfactorily performed in live animals. Bones with active red marrow must be selected and strict asepsis obtained. The site of puncture is shaved, thoroughly cleaned and infiltrated with local anesthetics. Stout needles15cm for cattle or horse and 2 cm for dog and cats should be used with 3.8% sterile sodium citrate drawn through it to prevent coagulation. Needle is inserted until bone is reached and is pushed into marrow cavity with a rotating motion. 0.5 ml of marrow is aspirated. *In cattle and horse external angle of the ileum* is used as puncture site and puncture is made in the middle of coxal tuber with needle directed towards the opposite hip joint. *Sternum* can also be used in cattle and *rib* in horse. In sheep 3rd sternebra is punctured with the animal sitting upright and penetration of bone should not exceed 0.5 cm. *Dog* is sampled from the *sternum* with animal on its back or from *external angle of ileum.*

Sample thus obtained can be treated in three ways. A drop of marrow is taken on a slide and smear slide prepared. Smears are fixed with methyl alcohol for 2 minutes and then stained with required stains. Samples may be washed in watch glass with 3.8% sodium citrate to get marrow flakes, place the flakes on slide along with a drop of serum then crush them with cover slips and prepare the smear which can be fixed and stained.

Liver Biopsy

It is useful in histological examinations and chemical estimation. It can be obtained from most animal species using specific trocar and cannula which is introduced into the liver high on the right side. *In cattle* puncture site is *11th intercostals space* about 15 cm below spinous process of corresponding vertebrae. *In horse it is 11th intercostals space or fourteenth intercostals space* on a line drawn from coxal tuber to the point of shoulder. *In dogs 8th to 10th intercostals space* is used as puncture site.

Lymph Node Biopsy

Whole lymph node can be removed by excising or using liver biopsy needles. Fine needle aspiration techniques are also desirable.

Skin Biopsy

It should be obtained from one or two representative skin lesions. It can be obtained by excision of diseased area or by means of punch biopsy. The area round the lesion is clipped, cleaned and infiltrated with local anesthetics avoiding the lesion. Lesion is either excised with scalpel or punched with a cylindrical hollow metal punch and wound closed with sutures. Both normal and abnormal tissue should be present in a sample which is placed in 10% formal saline. Biopsies for immuno-fluorescence studies are best cooled to –70^{0}c within 30 minutes of collection and not in formalin.

Muscles can be easily obtained with special needles. Kidney biopsy can be obtained by using keyhole surgery technique in dogs and cats.

3.12. Preputial Washings

The apparatus consists of 150ml flask, a flutter valve injection apparatus and a glass end-piece for insertion into the preputial orifice. The animal is restrained properly. The flask containing 100-150 ml of saline is placed for few minutes into hot water bath to raise the temperature of saline to 30-35°C. The glass end piece is placed well into the preputial orifice which is then held closely around the tube by digital pressure using the left hand. The container is raised and inverted so that saline floats into the preputial cavity. Prepuce is massaged vigorously so as to wash the mucous surfaces. Container is then lowered and fluid is massaged out of the prepuce back again in the container. Washing of the prepuce should neither have been made within previous seven days nor should the bull have been used for service or collection of semen. Clipping off the preputial hairs is usually unnecessary and the use of detergents is to be avoided.

3.13. Samples from Abortion Cases

In abortion cases fresh and clean placenta, uterine discharges on swabs in transport medium, fresh fetal stomach contents, fetal heart blood or cavity fluid, fetal lungs, kidney, liver should be collected and dispatched to the laboratory. The specimens are collected, packed separately and shipped conveniently in thermocool boxes with ice cubes or coolant packs or in dry ice with proper insulation. Fresh whole fetus is preferred.

Chapter 4

Culture, Isolation and Identification Techniques

SECTION-I

4.I.1. Culture and Isolation of Bacteria

Bacteria are small microorganisms, generally unicellular having relatively rigid cell walls that maintain their characteristic shape. Most of the bacteria are saprophytic or parasitic and only few are autotrophic. Bacteria grow on artificial, suitable nutrient, medium under appropriate conditions at a very rapid rate. Bacterial growth on artificial medium under-goes four phases.

(a) The Lag phase during which there is no significant multiplication of bacterial cells, however, they increase in size and exhibit increased metabolic rate. The length of this phase depends on the concentration of inoculum and cultural conditions.

(b) The Log phase *in* which cells divide at a constant rate by binary fission. There is linear relationship between logarithm of number of cells and time, with cells having high metabolic rate.

(c) The *Stationary phase* follows after rapid growth with decrease in the growth of bacterial cells until numbers of cells remain constant due to exhaustion of essential nutrients and accumulation of toxic waste products as a result of sugar fermentation in the medium.

(d) The *Decline phase* follows the stationary phase and the cells in culture start to die due to accumulation of toxic products of metabolism or autolysis.

Bacteria differ widely in the nutritional requirement and physical conditions needed for their growth. Majority of parasitic bacteria require organic nutrients like carbohydrates, amino acids, peptides or lipids to serve as source of carbon and energy. Growth factors like coenzymes, thiamine, riboflavin, nicotinic acid, pyridoxine, folic acid, biotin etc. are required for the growth in the medium. Oxygen and hydrogen can be supplied in water. Under appropriate suitable cultural conditions in the synthetic medium, the bacterial growth is linearly proportional to the concentration of growth factors and essential amino acids.

4.I.1.a. Culture Media

There are two broad groups of media, *liquid and solid medium*. Many liquid media or broths have been developed to favour the growth of most of bacteria. Liquid medium has limited utility in identification of species, however, necessary for biochemical tests of bacterial cultures. Organisms can not be separated from liquid bacterial mixed cultures. Solid media is of value in identification of bacteria by examining the colony characteristics and indispensable for the isolation of pure cultures from mixed cultures. Gelatin, coagulated serum or egg and agar can be used to solidify the media. However, agar is most commonly used for this purpose and remains un-melted at all incubation temperatures, besides being bacteriologically inert, with no growth promoting or inhibiting substances. Culture media are classified as under;

Defined synthetic medium is chemically defined medium prepared exclusively from pure chemical substances with known composition in distilled or deionised water and is useful for various experimental purposes.

Simple synthetic medium contains carbon and energy source like glucose or lactic acid, inorganic source of nitrogen usually in the form of ammonium chloride, phosphate or sulphate and various inorganic salts in buffered aqueous solution. This medium provides basic essentials for the growth of many non parasitic heterotrophs but does not favor growth of most of parasitic bacteria.

Complex synthetic medium is a simple synthetic medium enriched with certain amino acids, purines, pyrimidines and other growth factors, used for the growth of more exacting bacteria. They are prepared by the addition of substances like blood, serum or egg to the basal medium to meet the nutritional requirements of more exacting bacteria e.g. blood agar or broth, serum agar or broth.

Basal medium is a simple routine laboratory medium such as nutrient broth or peptone water. It is an aqueous extract of meat and digestion products of proteins, used for the growth of majority of pathogenic or commensal organisms of animals to be examined or investigated.

Selective medium favours the growth of a particular species while inhibiting the growth of others and is generally used to facilitate isolation of particular species of bacteria from mixed cultures e.g MacConkey's agar, Brilliant green agar, EMB agar, Deoxycholate agar, Selinite broth etc.

Indicator medium contain substances that are changed visibly as a result of metabolic activities of particular organisms.

4.I.1.b. Common Ingredients of Culture Medium

Water

Distilled or de-ionized or de-mineralized water must be used in preparation of culture medium.

Agar

Agar is derived from sea weeds containing mainly long chain polysaccharides, used at 1.5 to 3 % to solidify the culture medium. Agar is dissolved in any nutrient liquid medium if solid medium is desired. Agar along with nutrients which are not damaged by autoclaving are simultaneously dissolved and autoclaved, however, nutrients which are damaged in autoclaving are sterilized separately and then added to autoclaved agar when in liquid form and distributed in the required containers like petri dishes or in tubes as slants before it solidifies. Agar usually does not alter the pH of the medium to which it is added.

Peptone

It is a water soluble, golden powder with slightly acidic reaction, available commercially, obtained from lean meat or other protein material like heart muscles, casein, fibrin or soya by digestion with pepsin or trypsin. Peptone has ability to support the growth of moderately exacting bacteria.

Casein Hydrolysate

It largely consists of amino acids obtained by hydrolysis of the milk protein (casein) with hydrochloric acid or trypsin. Enzymatic hydrolysate contains full range of amino acids where as acid hydrolysate is nutritionally poor with decreased amino acid concentration. Since the composition of casein hydrolysate is fully known, it is added to minimal synthetic medium to render it suitable for growth of exacting bacteria

Meat Extract

It is derived from finely chopped lean beef held in boiling water for a short time when its readily soluble constituents pass into solution, which is then concentrated by evaporation. It contains water soluble protein degradation products like peptones, proteoses, amino acids, gelatin and other nitrogenous compounds like creatinine, creatin, purines etc. and accessory growth factors like thiamine, nicotinic acid, riboflavin, pyridoxine, pentothenic acid and choline.

Yeast Extract

It is prepared from washed cells of brewer's or baker's yeast, allowed to under go autolysis initiated by mild heating at 55^{0}C or in some cases hydrolysed with hydrochloric acid or enzymes. After removal of cell walls by centrifugation or filtration, extract is concentrated. It is supplied commercially as a powder, containing a wide range of amino-acids, growth factors especially of Vitamin B group and inorganic salts. It is mainly used as a source of growth factors and may be substituted for meat extract in culture medium.

Blood

Blood to be used in culture medium must be defibrinated (refer-3.1) and collected from rabbits, sheep or horses aseptically to exclude bacterial contamination, as its sterilization by heat would lead to its coagulation, denaturation and disintegration of cells. The defibrinated blood can be held in refrigerator for 2 months.

Serum

Serum collection does not necessarily require aseptic conditions as can be sterilized by Seitz filtration. Blood is collected preferably from sheep at abattoir and serum separated (refer-3.2).

4.I.2. Isolation of Pure Cultures from Mixed Cultures

It is obligatory to isolate the pertinent organism from a mixed culture before it is subjected to morphological, physiological, immunological or biochemical tests. This preliminary isolation is achieved by various techniques as described here under.

4.I.2.a. Platingout Technique

The mixed bacterial culture or infected material is smeared or rubbed thoroughly with the help of sterilized bacteriological loop over an area 'A'on a solid medium like nutrient or blood agar. The loop is again sterilized in a burner flame and two or three parallel lines are drawn from area 'A'on to the fresh surface of medium (B1,B2,B3).This procedure of drawing parallel lines from previously drawn lines on to a fresh surface with loop sterilized between each sequence is repeated as shown in figure. By this technique the bacteria are gradually diluted in each sequence of inoculating lines and are deposited singly at sufficient distance from each other. Each organism develops into a discrete colony on incubation, which is readily visible to the naked eye. Each colony constitutes a pure culture and should be picked up with the help of sterilized inoculating wire and subcultured in a fresh medium to obtain pure culture. While dealing with the small delicate colonies, extra care should be observed to eliminate the mixing, the use of low power binocular plate culture microscope may prove highly effective.

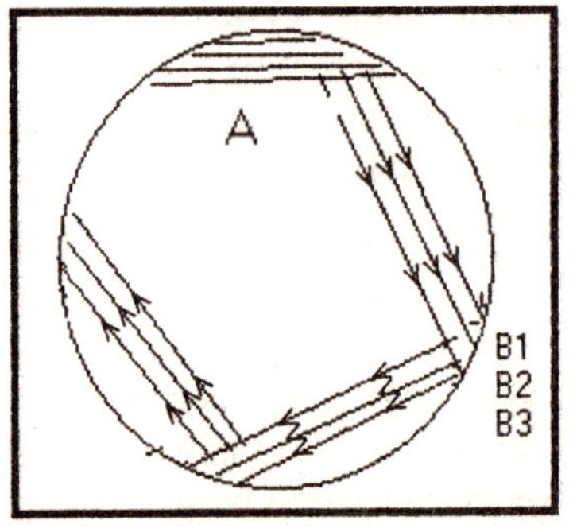

4.I.2.b. Plating Decimal Dilutions of the Inoculums

Series of tubes with melted agar are inoculated with decimal dilutions of mixed bacterial culture or infected material and then each tube poured out into separate petri dishes and allowed to solidify. The dishes are incubated and after incubation the colonies are distributed singly through out the solid medium. The single discrete colony should be picked up with the help of inoculating wire and subcultured in a fresh medium to obtain pure culture.

4.I.2.c. Heating and Subsequent Plating

This technique of isolating pure cultures from mixed ones is employed only in spore forming or heat resistant organisms. The mixed culture is heated in a water bath to 65°C for about 30 minutes sufficient to kill vegetative forms, leaving spores unaffected and after that the material is plated out on a solid agar medium and on incubation each spore will develop into an individual colony and can thus be isolated.

4.I.2.d. Use of Selective Medium

The use of selective medium favours the growth of one particular group of organisms and inhibits the growth of other organisms. There are many selective media available commercially for isolation of wide range of organisms such as Deoxycholate agar, Salmonella-Shigella agar, Tellurite medium etc.

4.I.2.e. Animal Inoculations

Laboratory animals are highly susceptible to certain organisms and are thus exploited for purifying the mixed cultures. When the laboratory animals are inoculated with mixed culture, they die of a particular disease and the causative organisms can be isolated from the heart blood in a pure form such as mice is used to isolate the pasturella from mixed cultures or guinea pigs for isolating tubercle bacillus or clostridium.

4.I.3. Cultural Conditions

Incubation of bacterial cultures is carried out at 37-38°C for 24 to 48 hours in most of the cases, however, incubation may be as long as a week in certain organisms. It is important to note that the plates are incubated in inverted position after being inoculated, marked and labeled preferably on the portion containing medium. However the gelatin plates are not incubated in inverted position because some organisms may liquefy the gelatin and will lead to loss of medium and culture.

Growth of the *aerobic organisms* does not involve any special methods of incubation but culture of anaerobic organisms requires specific cultural conditions that establish anaerobiasis.

Simplest method for culture of *anaerobic organisms* is to grow the organisms deep in solid media like agar tubes. Addition of glucose at 0.5% concentration renders it anaerobic because of acting as reducing agent. Tubes can be inoculated deep by long straight inoculating wire or agar can be melted, cooled to 45^{0}C and charged with inoculum, mixed by rotation and allowed to solidify before incubation. Semisolid agar medium (nutrient broth added with 1/ 10th of 2% nutrient agar) enriched with glucose 0.5% or sodium thioglucolate 0.1% or ascorbic acid 0.1% can be conveniently used as culture medium for anaerobes.

Glucose broth can be rendered completely anaerobic by keeping it in boiling water for 5 minutes and then added sterile melted petroleum jelly that seals the medium from air when cooled.

Robertson's cooked meat medium is very useful for anaerobic work. Sterilized muscle tissue contains reducing substances, thus is effective in maintaining anaerobic conditions at the bottom of tubes.

However to grow anaerobes on the surface of the solid medium, it is necessary to provide anaerobic conditions, that can be achieved bv use of anaerobic systems available with certain companies like HiMedia.

Organisms which require carbon dioxide for their growth in medium such as Brucella, Meningococci, Gonococci, Pneumococci etc. can be conveniently cultured while incubating in carbon dioxide incubators.

4.I.4. Preservation of Cultures

Bacteria display great variation in their ability to remain alive in the culture. Some species are poorly viable and their cultures die out within few days, irrespective of storage conditions eg. Neisseria species, thus its preservation demands its subculturing every 3-4 days. Contrary to it spore forming species remain viable for years together and need not to be sub- cultured oftenly. Where as some non sporing species remain viable for months or even years under suitable conditions like Enterobacteriacae which can be preserved in Coagulated egg medium at room temperature or refrigeration temperature. Cultures can be preserved in agar tubes when cultured as stabs and covered with sterilized mineral oil before being sealed with wax plugging.

Bacterial cultures, or anti sera can conveniently be preserved for several years by freeze drying procedure when cultures are suspended in nutrient broth containing 1% peptone and beef or meat extract. Many other media have been used successfully for lyophilization but most generally recommended is serum broth containing 7.5% glucose (one volume of nutrient broth with 30% glucose + three volumes of sterile inactivated serum).

4.I.5. Disposal of Cultures

Disposal of cultures in the laboratory is of paramount importance because any carelessness in disposing the cultures may put laboratory personnel as well as other cultures to a great risk of infection and contamination. It is better to kill the cultures to be discarded by heat treatment or antiseptics or disinfectants (refer 1.2) before it is drained out or its containers are washed. All the tubes, Petri dishes, glass slides, plugs, culture bottles or lids should be emmersed in 3% Lysol or cresol in a wash tub. Cultures of tubercle bacillus or spore forming organisms must be killed by autoclaving.

4.I.6. Identification of Bacteria

Identification of microbes involves a series of laboratory procedures and tests.

1. In the first instance culture on solid medium, provides a tract for identifying organisms through examination of colony characteristics by naked eye or hand lens.
2. Further clue in identification of organisms is provided by staining techniques of fixed cultures or infected materials (refer 4.I.6.a.) or examination of moist preparations (unstained material suspended in a small drop of water or broth on a clean glass slide with a cover slip placed over it).
3. Determination of motility by hanging drop method (place a drop of culture in the middle of clean glass cover slip with out spreading it and place a cavity slide carefully over the coverglass. It will be better to use drops of wax or Vaseline on the corners of the concavity of a cavity slide. The slide with adhering cover glass is picked up and quickly turned over and examined under microscope).

   However the most reliable method for identification of organisms still remains its biochemical characteristics. Credibility of identification of a culture by its biochemical parameters depend largely on the use of pure cultures in the test medium.

4.I.6.a. Staining Methods

Staining is generally employed to study the morphological and staining characters of the organism. The microbial colony on solid media is taken with the help of bacteriological loop or wire and mixed with a drop of distilled water on a clean slide. It is spread on the slide and air dried. Culture from liquid media is taken as a film loop of culture on to the slide, spread and air dried. When the smear is dry, fix it by passing the slide through flame two to three times avoiding over heating and cooled before staining. Fixing of smears like blood smears can be achieved with methyl alcohol. Some important staining methods commonly used in staining of films in the laboratory are detailed as under.

Gram's Staining

This is the most important and commonly employed staining method in bacteriology. Certain bacteria are stained with dyes like methyl violet, crystal violet or gentian violet and then with iodine, that fixes the stain in the cells. The stain can not be removed by decolorizing agents like alcohol or acetone and such organisms that retain the stain are called Gram positive organisms while others that get decolorized completely and take counter-stain are referred as Gram negative organisms. Gram positive organisms are dark violet in colour and are easily distinguished from Gram negative organisms which stain pink.

Procedure

1. Make a smear on slide as referred above and cover the whole slide with methyl violet stain. Allow stain to remain on the slide for 2 to 3 minutes.
2. Pour off the methyl violet stain and wash off the excess stain by Grams iodine solution by holding the slide at a steep slope.
3. Cover the whole slide with iodine solution and allow the stain to remain on slide for 2 minutes.
4. Pour off the stain from the slide and decolourize with acetone or alcohol or supplied decolourizer. The slide is held at slope

and decolourizer is poured from the upper end of the slide so as to cover whole slide and this process is completed within 30 seconds.

5. Wash the slide thoroughly with the tap water.
6. Flood the whole slide with basic fuchsin stain and allow it to remain for 1 to 2 minutes.
7. Wash thoroughly the slide under running tap water. Blot and dry the slide in air.
8. Examine the smear under oil immersion, gram positive organisms are violet and gram negative are pink in colour.

Ziel-Neelsen Staining

This staining method is employed to identify acid fast bacteria like tubercle bacillus. Ordinary dye does not penetrate the substance of bacillus, hence basic fuchsin with phenol is used to stain the tubercle bacillus while applying the heat. Any strong acid is used as decolorizer.

Procedure

1. Prepare the slide smear as referred above.
2. Cover the slide with strong carbol fuchsin added with phenol 5% in solution and heat the slide until steam rises.
3. Allow the stain to remain on slide for 5 minutes and keep the stain hot by applying heat to the slide, but do not allow it to evaporate or dry and if necessary add more stain to keep slide flooded with stain.
4. Wash slide with water.
5. Cover the slide with 20% sulphuric acid or acid alcohol (3ml conc. hydrochloric acid + 97ml of 95% alcohol) for about a minute. Wash the slide with water and pour more acid on the slide and repeat this process several times. Decolourization is completed when film gives a faint pink colour after washing.
6. Wash the slide thoroughly with water.
7. Counter stain with methylene blue or dilute malachite green for ½ to 1 minute.
8. Wash the slide in water, blot and dry the slide.

9. Examine the slide under oil immersion. Acid fast organisms stain bright red while as other cells stain blue or green according to counter stain.

Methylene Blue Staining

Loffler;s methylene blue is the most generally used stain(30% methylene blue in 0.01% aqueous KOH solution). It is a very good stain to use when studying the morphology of organisms. Oftenly used in staining diphtheria bacilli and pasturella species.

Procedure

1. Make thin smear of material or culture to be examined on a slide, dry it in air and fix with gentle heat.
2. Cover the smear with stain and allow it to stand for 3 minutes, heat slightly if deep staining is desired.
3. Wash the slide under tap water. Blot and dry and examine under oil immersion.

Neisser's Methylene Blue Staining

This staining method gives better results in identification of metachromatic granules of corynebacterium that take deep blue colour and remainder of organism as pink. Neisser's methylene blue stain comprises of 1gm methylene blue + 50ml ethyl alcohol + 50ml glacial acetic acid + 1 litre distilled water.

Procedure

1. Make thin smear of material or culture to be examined on a slide, dry it in air and fix with gentle heat.
2. Cover the smear with stain and allow it to stand for 3 minutes.
3. Wash off the stain with diluted 1 in 10 iodine solution(1% iodine + 2% potassium iodide). Leave the iodine solution on the smear for a minute.
4. Wash the slide under tap water and counter stain with neutral red solution(1g neutral red + 2ml of 1% acetic acid + 1000ml distilled water) for 3 minutes.
5. Wash the slide in water and dry. Examine the slide under oil immersion.

Nigrosin Staining Method

Nigrosin staining is a simplest method of staining for making preliminary examination of a culture to show shape, size and arrangement of organisms. It is prepared as 10 % solution of nigrosin in water added with 0.5% formalin as preservative.

Procedure

1. Place a drop of nigrosin stain on the slide, mix it with the culture to be studied with the help of a loop.
2. Make the smear on the same slide or on another with the help of a loop.
3. Dry and examine the slide under oil immersion.

Staining of Spores

Spores are not demonstrated by the simple staining methods, special methods are hence employed for examination of spores in the organisms.

Acid Fast Staining for Spores

This method of staining is same as referred above except that counter staining is done with 1% aqueous methylene blue for 3 minutes. The spores are stained bright red and protoplasm of organism as blue.

Melachite Green Staining for Spores

1. Make thin smear of material or culture to be examined on a slide, dry it in air and fix with gentle heat.
2. Place the slide on the rim of a beaker of boiling water with film uppermost.
3. When water droplets have condensed on the under surface of the slide, flood it with 5% aqueous solution of malachite green and allow stain to remain on slide for a minute.
4. Wash the slide in cold water.
5. Flood the slide with 0.5% safranine or 0.05% basic fuchsin for half a minute.
6. Wash , blot and dry.
7. Microscopic examination reveals green spores in red organism.

Staining of Capsules

The capsules of the organisms present in animal tissues, fluids or pus can clearly be demonstrated by common staining like Gram's staining, methylene blue staining, Leishman's staining. However staining of cultures for demonstration of capsules requires special staining methods. The best method of staining the organisms from liquid or solid medium for demonstration of capsules is Wet Film India Ink Method.

Procedure

1. Place a loopful of India ink on a clean microscopic slide as a drop of ink.
2. Mix a small portion of culture material from solid medium or a loop of culture from a liquid medium with the ink on the slide.
3. Place a clean cover slip on the drop and press it firmly so as to obtain a thin film.
4. Examine under oil immersion preferably under phase contrast microscope for capsule. A clear space that lies between highly refractile surface membrane of organism and the dark back ground of ink particles represents capsule. The non- capsulated organisms do not display this clear zone.

Fontana's Staining

This method of staining is widely employed in the demonstration of spirochaetes in films. It requires a fixative(1ml acetic acid + 2ml formalin + 100ml distilled water), a mordant (1g phenol + 5g tannic acid + 100ml distilled water)and an ammoniated silver nitrate (add 10% ammonia to 0.5% aqueous solution of silver nitrate until precipitate formed gets dissolved and add more silver nitrate drop by drop until precipitate returns and does not re-dissolve).

Procedure

1. Fix the film thrice with the fixative for 30 seconds each time.
2. Wash with absolute alcohol and allow alcohol to stand for 3 minutes.
3. Pour off the alcohol and burn off the remainder carefully until the film is dry.

4. Cover with the mordant and apply heat till steam arises and allow it to stand for 30 seconds.
5. Wash the film with distilled water and dry it.
6. Cover with ammoniated silver nitrate, apply heat till steam arises and allow it to remain on slide for 30 seconds, when film becomes brown in colour.
7. Wash the film with distilled water and dry the slide before mounting in Canada balsam under coverslip.
8. Examine the mounted slide; the spirochaetes are stained brownish black on a brownish yellow back ground.

Castaneda's Staining

The study of rickettsiae is facilitated with the Castaneda's staining besides Giemsa's. This staining requires 1N HCl, formaldehyde buffer(40ml formalin neutralized with 1N NaOH + 960ml phosphate buffer pH 7.2), 1%Azur II and 0.25% safranine.

Procedure

1. Fix the film in 1 N HCl for 2 minutes.
2. Wash the film with distilled water.
3. Cover the slide with diluted Azur II (1 in 10 formaldehyde buffer) and allow it stand for 20 minutes.
4. Wash the slide with distilled water thoroughly.
5. Counter-stain with 0.25% safranine for 10 seconds.
6. Wash in running water, blot and dry the slide.
7. Examine under oil immersion when rickettsiae stain blue protoplasm and red nuclei.

Giemsa's Staining

This staining method gives the best results for demonstration of spirochetes and certain protozoa, besides it is useful in demonstration of rickettsia and virus inclusion bodies.

Procedure

1. Make thin smear of blood or culture to be examined on a slide, dry it in air and fix in absolute methyl alcohol for 15 minutes.
2. Stain the slide in a coplin jar with one part of stain and ten

parts of buffer solution pH 7.0 for 1 hour to 3 hours.

3. Wash the slide with buffer and dry in air before examining under oil immersion.

4.I.6.b. Biochemical Tests

A wide range of tests are there to identify microorganisms such as fermentation of carbohydrates; splitting of proteins, aminoacids; changes in single radicals etc. Some important tests are discussed here under.

Liquefaction of Gelatin and Coagulated Serum

Proteolytic activity of organisms is usually studied by inoculation in gelatin medium (gelatin-12%+beef extract-0.3%+peptone-0.5% in distilled water, pH-7 and autoclaved after dispensing in tubes at 121°C for 15 minutes).

1. Stab culture of the pure organism is made in the gelatin medium.
2. Incubation is carried out at 37°C for one or more days.
3. Tubes are placed in a refrigerator to observe liquefaction.

Indol test

Indol is produced from tryptophane and any medium used for this test should contain tryptophane in significant quantity. Indol is then tested for by reaction with para dimethyleaminobenzaldehyde.

1. Inoculate the test organism in basal medium (peptone-2% + sod.chloride-0.5% in distilled water, pH-7.4 and autoclaved)
2. Incubate the medium for 48 to 96 hours at 37°C.
3. Add 0.5ml of Kovac's reagent and shake gently.
4. Development of red colour indicates positive reaction.

Reduction of Nitrates

This test determines the presence of an enzyme nitrate reductase.

1. Inoculate the test culture in medium (potassium nitrate-0.02% + peptone-0.5% in distilled water).
2. Incubate the medium for 96 hours at 37°C.

3. Add 0.1ml of test reagent (equal volumes of sulphanilic acid-0.8% in 5N acetic acid + Alpha-naphthylamine-0.5% in 5N acetic acid).
4. Development of red colour within few minutes labels the test nitrate reduction positive.

Methyl Red Test

It is applied to detect the production of acid during glucose fermentation.

1. Inoculate 5-10ml tube with MR-VP medium or glucose peptone water (peptone-0.5% + K_2Po_4- 0.5%, autoclave and add sterilized glucose to a conc.Of 0.5%).
2. Incubate the tubes at 37°C for 48 hours.
3. Add about few drops of methyl red indicator (0.02% soln.of methyl red in 95% alcohol).
4. Red colour indicates positive and yellow negative.

Voges-Proskauer Test

It is conducted for the detection of acetyl methyl carbinol,an intermediate breakdown product of glucose.

1. Inoculate 10ml of MR-VP medium or glucose peptone water as in M.R.test.
2. Incubate the medium at 37°C for 48 hours.
3. Add to it 3ml of 5% alpha naphthol in absolute ethanol and 1ml of 40%sodium hydroxide.
4. Shake well and watch for pink colour in 5-10 minutes which should deepen with time in positive case.

Hydrogen Sulphide Test

Some organisms produce hydrogen sulphide from sulphur containing aminoacids which is demonstrated by its ability to form black insoluble ferrous salt.

1. Inoculate the tubes with medium(meat extract-0.75% + peptone-2.5% + sod.chloride -0.5% + gelatin- 12% in distilled water, pH-7.6, sterilize in free steam for 10-20 minutes, cool to 55°C and add 5ml of 10% fresh ferrous chloride, filter sterilized).

2. Incubate the medium at 20°C for minimum 7 days.
3. Observe the blackening of medium daily in positive cases.
4. This medium also tests gelatin liquefaction.

Another satisfactory method is the use of 5 x 50mm filter paper strips.

1. Soak the strips in a saturated solution of lead acetate.
2. Dry the strips in a Petri plate placed in hot air oven for 1 hour
3. Use a broth or solid medium, preferably infusion broth.
4. Insert one strip in to the tube so that one-half projects below the plug, just after inoculation.
5. Observe the strip for blackening during incubation.

Oxidase Test

1. Prepare 1% solution of tetra-methyl-para-phenylene diamine hydrochloride in distilled water.
2. Keep the solution in a corked bottle and use it only for a week and not beyond that.
3. Pour the prepared dye over the growth on a suitable solid medium to cover the surface and immediately decanted.
4. In positive case organisms will rapidly develop a purple colour.
5. It shall be better not to use whole plate but a colony on loop is satisfactory that can be covered with the dye.

Presently strips are also available which have shelf life of few months in air tight bottles at room temperature. They can be prepared by soaking filter paper strips in 1% solution of freshly prepared tetramethyl-para-phenylene-diamine and then freeze dried. The strips will have light purple tint.

1. Take a strip moisten it in a Petri dish.
2. Smear the colony to be tested over the moist area
3. Positive reaction is indicated by development of deep purple hue within seconds.

Citrate Utilization Test

1. Inoculate the Koser's citrate broth or Simmon's citrate agar.
2. Incubate for 2-5 days at 37°C.
3. Turbidity/growth in Koser broth and blue colour in Simmon's agar indicate citrate utilization.

Urease Test

1. Inoculate a loopful of agar culture of test organism to 1ml of urea broth (KH_2PO_4-3.64g + Na_2HPO_4-3.8g + Urea-8g + yeast extract-40mg + 0.02%phenol red-20ml + distilled water-380ml, pH-6.8, filter sterilization) in a small tube.
2. Observe in half an hour for a pink to red colour indicating urea decomposition.

Coagulase Test

1. Dilute rabbit or human citrated plasma 1:4 with saline.
2. Mix a loopful of test culture with 0.5ml of plasma.
3. Incubate at 37°C for about 4 hours.
4. Observe for coagulum.
5. Any amount of coagulation labels the test positive.

Sugar Tests

Bacteria do have ability to metabolize carbohydrates for its energy by fermentation or oxidation and differ greatly in this character. Metabolism of sugars results in the production of acids and gas. This ability of organisms is being exploited in identification of organisms while conducting sugar tests which broadly involves four steps;

Growth in Suitable Medium

The organism to be tested is grown in a suitable basal medium. The most commonly used media are;

(a) Peptone water base – peptone : 1%, sod. chloride: 0.5% in distilled water and pH adjusted to 7.2-7.3.

(b) Broth base – meat extract: 0.5%, peptone: 1%, sod. chloride: 0.3%, Na_2HPO_4 : 0.2% in distilled water.

(c) Serum water – sheep or ox serum: 33% in distilled water or 0.1% peptone water.

Preparation of Indicator

Phenol Red

1. Prepare 0.2% solution (dissolving 1g phenol red + 10ml 0.1N NaOH + 10ml 0.1N HCl + distilled water to make 500ml).
2. Add this indicator to the basal medium to achieve 5% concentration of it in medium.

Bromothymol Blue

1. Prepare 0.2% solution (1g bromothymol blue + 25ml 0.1 N NaOH + 475ml distilled water).
2. Add this indicator to the basal medium to achieve 0.12% concentration in the medium.

Preparation of Test Sugar

1. Prepare 10% solution of fermentable sugar to be used for test.
2. Sterilize it by tyndallization or filtration (described in chapter I).
3. Use the sugar in the basal medium in an amount to get 1% concentration of sugar in the medium.

Insertion of Durham's Fermentation Tube in the Medium

Procedure

1. Prepare the desired basal medium.
2. Add the indicator as referred above.
3. Dispense the medium in tubes in 5ml volumes.
4. Insert Durham's fermentation tube in each tube.
5. Stopper the tubes with cotton wool.
6. Autoclave the tubes with medium and fermentation tube at 121°C for 10 minutes.
7. Add test sugar (10%) at 0.25ml in each tube.
8. Inoculate the medium with a loopful of pure test culture.
9. Incubate the tubes at 37°C for 24 hours generally. Incubation period may be even days in late fermenters.
10. Observe for change in colour to yellow and gas formation in Durham's tube.
11. Change in colour indicates acid formation while gas in tube indicates fermentation with production of gas.

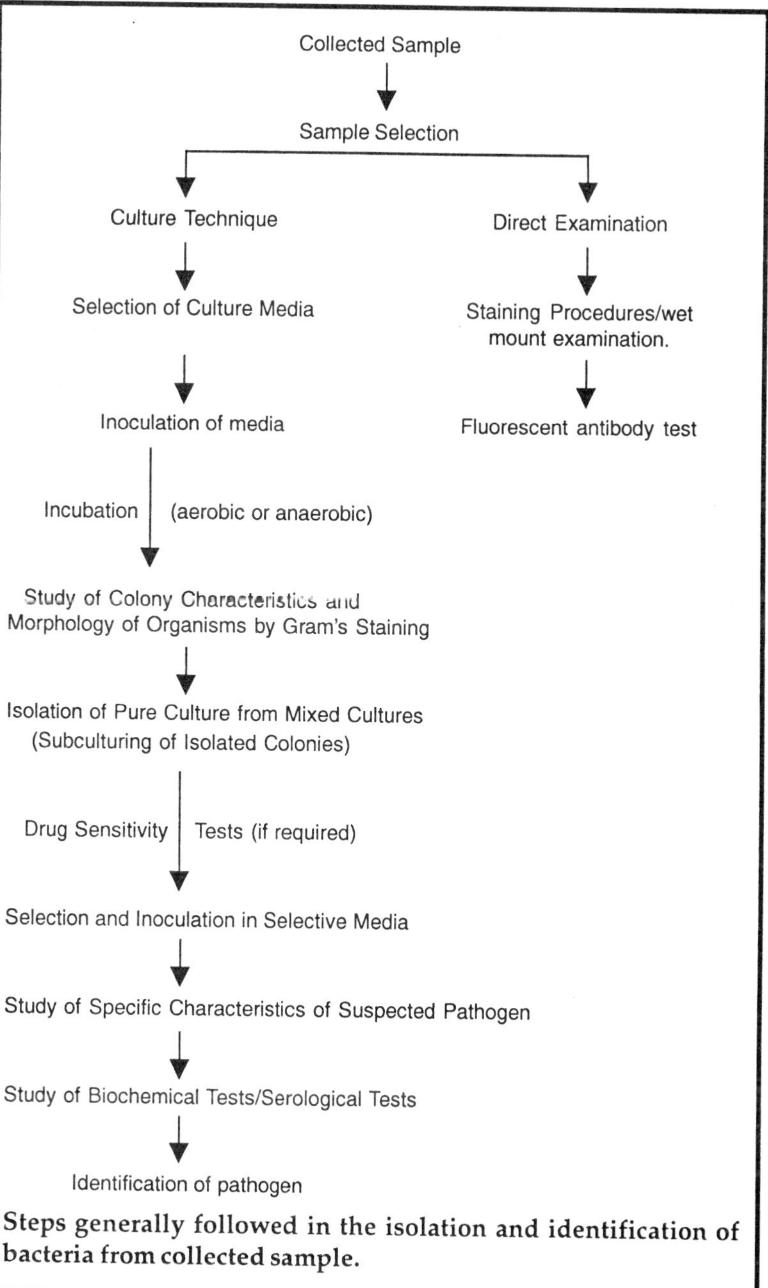

Steps generally followed in the isolation and identification of bacteria from collected sample.

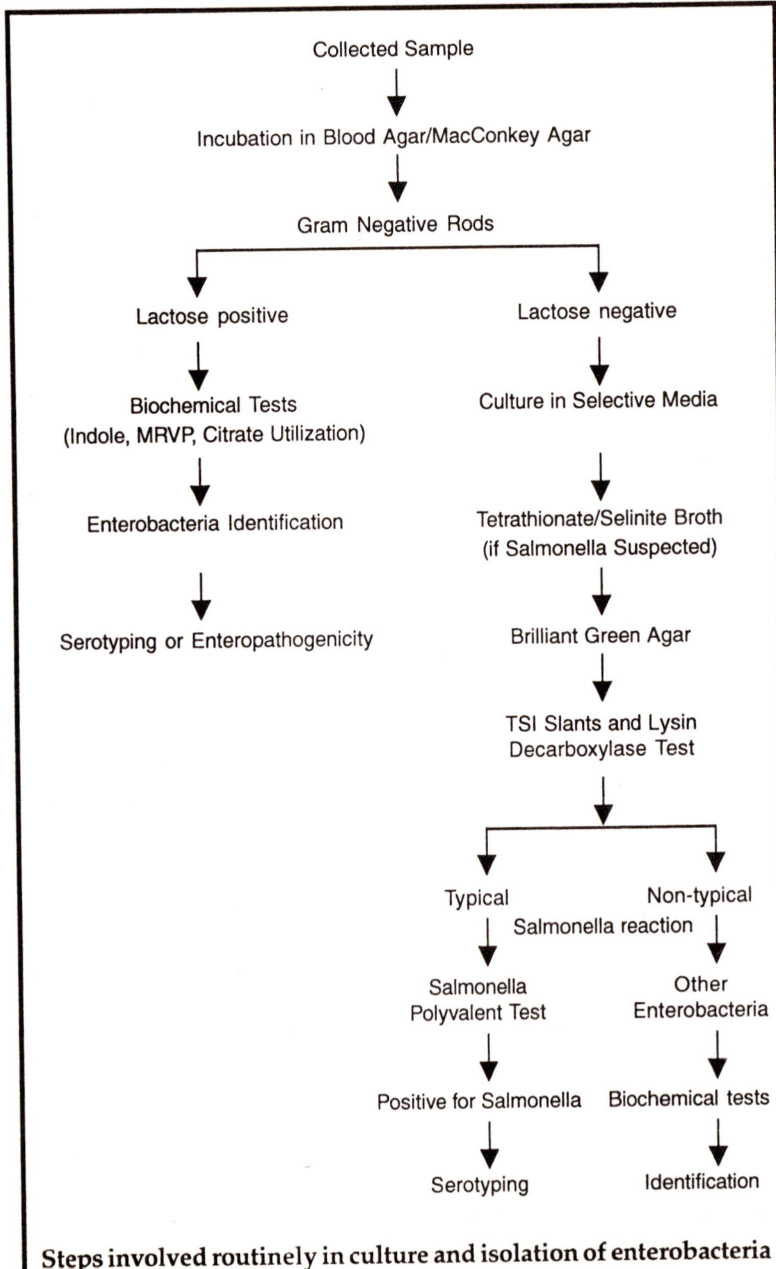

Steps involved routinely in culture and isolation of enterobacteria

SECTION-II

4.II.1. Culture and Isolation of Fungi

The majority of diseases caused by pathogenic fungi and yeasts are those which produce superficial lesions of the skin and mucous membranes like Microsporum, Trichophyton and Epidermophyton. Diseases like pulmonary and intestinal actinomycosis or aspergillosis or cryptococcosis are less frequently recognized clinically with out producing any local lesions and diagnosis of such infections is most often delayed or discovered only at necropsy. However, cultural methods are frequently the only means of isolation and identification of fungi. Animal inoculations are also some times useful.

The diagnosis of fungal infections broadly involves following laboratory procedures.

1. Wet mount examination of tissues or mucous containing specimens in 10% potassium hydroxide that permits visualization of fungi.
2. Wet mount examination of teased portions from fungal colonies stained with lactophenol cotton blue.
3. Staining of tissue sections and clinical material with periodic acid-schiff (PAS) or methenamine silver stains.
4. Culture in Sabouraud's glucose agar containing antibiotics like chloramphenicol.
5. Culture in Brain heart infusion agar or blood agar which in fact favours the growth of yeast phase of dimorphic fungi when incubation is carried for a week or more.
6. Slide culture and then wet mount examination.

The material collected aseptically should be transferred in to the culture medium immediately to eliminate contamination. Specimens from deep mycosis should routinely be cultured in an aerobic blood agar at 37°C and on two Sabouraud's glucose or maltose agar plates keeping one at room temperature and other at 37°C. Hairs, skin scrapings should be rubbed over the surface of culture medium plates by means of forceps and then inserted into cuts made in the medium. These materials are likely to contain contaminating bacteria that can be eliminated by storing the material in paper envelops for one or more weeks or immersed in 70% ethyl alcohol for 2-3 minutes.

Culture of sputum is advised to be done on two plates of Sabouraud's glucose agar and two plates of blood agar containing 30iu penicillin and 30ug of streptomycin per ml. One plate of each is incubated at 37°C and other at room temperature. Dry swabs can be inoculated in Sabouraud's broth and then subcultured on plates.

Cultures should be examined every 2 to 3 days. Yeasts, actinomyces, nocardia and candida grow comparatively rapidly within 2 to 5 days where- as blastomyces, coccidiodes and histoplasma grow slowly in 5 to 8 days and ringworm fungi take 2 to 3 weeks for development of colony. To obtain a pure culture, material should be taken from near the edge of the colony and subcultured in a fresh medium. The texture and colour of colony should be observed on both its upper and lower sides and any diffusible pigment entering into the medium should be recorded.

4.II.2. Identification of Fungi

Materials collected for mycological evaluation should be divided into three parts, one for direct microscopic examination, second for cultural isolation and third for animal inoculation or other special tests.

4.II.2.a. Direct Examination

Direct examination of material is sufficient for diagnosis of fungus in many instances, however, it does not suffice for the identification of species. The scrapings or hairs are put on a clean slide and treated with a drop of 10% solution of potassium hydroxide under a cover slip for 5 to 10 minutes. Slide is passed through a burner flame 3 to 4 times and then examined under microscope. Staining of fungi is seldom practiced in superficial mycosis because the hydroxide quickly decolorizes the most stains. Lactophenol cotton blue stain is, however, the best stain for demonstration of fungi in wet or dry preparations.

4.II.2.b. Microscopic Examination of Wet Mounts

Microscopic examination of wet mounts from specimens of skin scrapings, hairs, pus or exudates is the first step in establishing fungal infections. The microscopic examination of culture is carried out by removing some sporing mycelium on the point of an inoculating wire(needle mount) and transferred into a drop of lactophenol blue stain on a microscopic slide and teased out.

Coverslip is applied and excess stain is drained by pressing down the coverslip gently under blotting paper. Microscopic examination should be focused on microconidia, macroconidia, chlamydospores besides vegetative hyphae.

4.II.2.c. Slide Culture Method for Identification of Fungi

For easy identification fungus can be subcultured on an agar block of 2mm thickness held between a slide and coverslip. This method of culture enables the undisturbed observation of growth at various stages during course of culture. Inoculation is made by a needle tip of culture into the agar block at four edges. Incubation is carried out at room temperature in a sealed jar with some water or soaked blotting paper at its bottom to avoid desiccation. Slide is examined every day or two for growth under microscope. When sufficient growth develops, discard the agar block carefully without disturbing the growth on slide or coverslip. Apply a drop of 95% ethyl alcohol to the growth on slide or coverslip and allow it to evaporate, then add a drop of lactophenol blue stain and gently place coverslip on slide. After overnight standing excess stain is blotted out from the edges of the coverslip and microscopic examination is carried out for identification of fungi.

4.II.2.c. Staining of Fungi

Fungi are demonstrated under microscope as a wet needle mount and most commonly stained with lacto-phenol cotton blue (20g phenol crystals + 20ml lactic acid + 40ml glycerol + 20ml distilled water + 50mg cotton blue or methyl blue). Dissolve the phenol crystals in warm liquids before adding dye.

Procedure

1. Place a drop of stain on a clean slide.
2. Mix gently a fragment of culture taken with a needle (needle mount).
3. Cover it with a cover slip, apply little pressure and avoid trapping of air bubbles.
4. Examine under microscope.

The slide culture preparations of fungi are stained and studied undisturbed while applying a drop of stain and mounted under microscope.

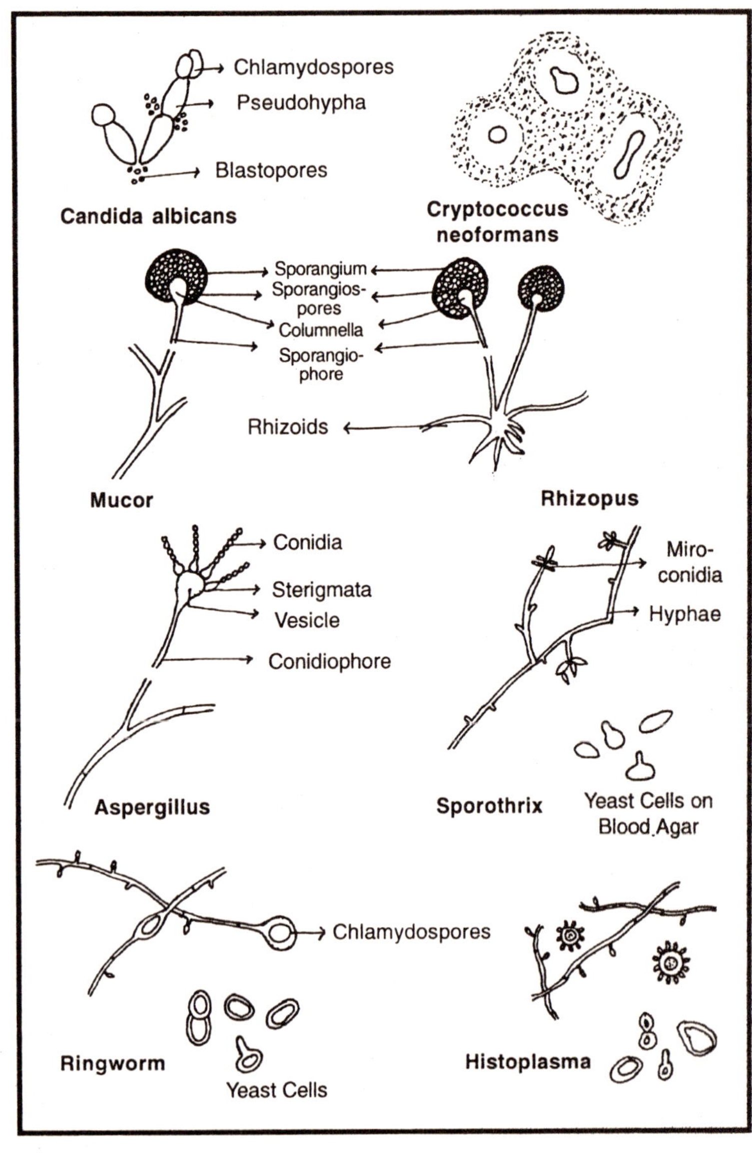
Chlamydospores
Pseudohypha
Blastopores
Candida albicans
Cryptococcus neoformans
Sporangium
Sporangiospores
Columnella
Sporangiophore
Rhizoids
Mucor
Rhizopus
Conidia
Sterigmata
Vesicle
Conidiophore
Aspergillus
Miro-conidia
Hyphae
Sporothrix
Yeast Cells on Blood.Agar
Chlamydospores
Ringworm
Yeast Cells
Histoplasma

SECTION- III

4.III.1. Culture and Isolation of Viruses

Viruses are very small in size, measured in millimicrones, largest viruses are half the size of smallest bacteria. They grow only in living cells, resist action of antibiotics and other agents that destroy bacteria, contain only one type of nucleic acid, multiply by a complex process and not by binary fission and are covered by a protein coat called capsid. The capsid is formed of number of capsomeres and enclosed by a membrane through which protrude a large number of projections in which resides the enzyme that confers hemagglutination property of certain viruses.

Viruses replicate in living cells only. Most of viruses can be grown in cell/tissue culture systems, embryonated eggs or laboratory animals.

4.III.1.a. Animal Tissue Culture Techniques

The animal tissue culture or cell culture techniques have founded a new edifice in the area of biotechnology research. Besides virus culture, mechanism of action at molecular level of drugs, hormones etc can be evaluated with ease using cell lines. Cell lines can be used in diagnosis of various disease conditions by propagating and isolating the causative agent (virus) in cell cultures in vitro. The prime function of the organ, tissue or cell culture systems is to reproduce the in-vivo conditions for normal cells to be grown in chemically defined medium. It is of paramount importance to provide completely sterile environment in maintaining cell lines. Introduction of antibiotics and antifungal substances in cell cultures besides use of laminar flow hoods, sterile gloves, masks are helpful in limiting the contamination of cultures. Cell cultures are preferred over egg or animal inoculation because cell cultures can be produced in large quantities and stored at -70°C, besides they give a clear cytopathic effect and can be radiolabelled to study the details of virus multiplication. The techniques of maintaining and propagating tissues, cells and cell lines under sterile conditions, used for virus propagation or conducting biomedical research, can be categorized into three types.

Organ Culture

This consists primarily of organ pieces or explants maintained under sterile conditions such as respiratory or intestinal epithelium. It is basically suitable for conducting studies on cellular differentiation since the cultured tissue has limited life span.

Cell Culture (Primary Monolayer)

For almost all diagnostic and research work, monolayer cell cultures are used. Cells are obtained following enzymatic dissociation of organs or tissues like Kidney, testis, thyroid etc. and then maintained in chemically defined tissue culture medium. Trypsin is used for cell dispersion and embryonic cells are often used because they grow well and are easily dissociated. The dissociated cells are suspended in growth medium contained in cell/tissue culture bottles, in which the cells get adhered to the bottom, they flatten and repeatedly divide until a confluent sheet of cells is formed. The monolayer cell cultures in vitro differentiate into three basic morphological types;

(a) Epithelial polyhedral cells derived from ectodermal and endodermal tissues like renal cortex, thyroid, amnion and epidermis.

(b) Fibroblast-spindle shaped cells derived from mesodermal tissue like connective tissue, embryonic muscle.

(c) Macrophages derived from macrophages and monocytes, difficult to grow as secondary cultures.

Secondary cultures are produced by dispersion of these primary cell layers by trypsin and EDTA mixture and seeded in fresh tissue culture medium. Primary cell cultures have limitations and after several passages cells stop to grow.

Continuous Cell Cultures

However, cell lines have been developed which can be passaged indefinitely, referred as continuous established cell lines which are essentially derived from natural mutation or retroviral transformation of normal cells of a particular organ which have the property of immortality. Established cell line culture is preferred over other cell cultures because of being capable of withstanding freezing and then reviving such as Michigan Cancer Foundation -7 (MCF-7), Epithelial Human Breast Adenocarcinoma, Human Hepatoma (Hep-G-2), African Green Monkey Kidney Cells(Vero-C-1008), Fibroblasts, Hela cell line etc. Continuous cell cultures are mostly used in virus work but primary cultures are still used to isolate some viruses because primary cultures are thought to be more susceptible to infection.

Suspension Cultures

Suspension cultures are used where large scale production of the virus is required as in the case of vaccine production or for biomedical studies. Some cell lines are adopted to grow in suspension where medium is continuously stirred and aerated. Suspension cell cultures have also been grown from viral and non-viral tumors like lymphoid tumers of Marek's disease, bovine leucosis.

Maintenance and Cryopreservation of Cell Lines

It is essential to maintain the cell lines in completely sterile conditions because they can get contaminated very easily with bacteria, viruses or fungi and there is practically no possibility to correct this problem and the only choice is to discard the culture. The cell lines are maintained and propagated in chemically defined medium such as TCM-199, MEM, RPMI-1640 etc. The common ingredients are amino-acids, vitamins, glucose, sodium chloride and buffers along with antibiotics such as penicillin and streptomycin. Cell lines do require foetal calf serum usually 7 to 10%, to ensure normal growth, in the medium.

Cryopreservation of cell lines can be achieved either in computer driven equipments or using specialized procedures involving cryoprotectants like glycerol or dimethyl-sulphoxide. The storage of cells is carried in liquid nitrogen at -196°C. and these cells can be retrieved, revived and propagated like normal cells at will.

4.III.1.b. Animal Inoculation Method

Experimental animals are being exploited for virus culture, isolation besides virus attenuation, raising of monoclonal or polyclonal antibodies and study of pathogenicity and host immune reactions. The natural host is still being used in evaluation of pathogenesis, immunology, vaccine trials, diagnosis and chemotherapy. The experimental animal used should be pathogen free with no prior immunity to particular virus. The experimental animals in case of animal viruses may be homologous or heterologous hosts. The most frequently used are laboratory animals like rabbit, guinea pig, mice or ferrets.

4.III.1.c. Embryonated Egg Inoculation Method

The use of experimental animal in virus work has been replaced to a great extent by inoculation of live embryonated chicken eggs. Chicken embryos are used in culture and isolation of many avian and few mammalian viruses. This method is more feasible, economical and needs less expertise than cell culture and animal inoculation. The route of embryo inoculation differs with viruses to be isolated and the inoculation technique is described in detail in chapter 6. The presence of virus in embryo can be detected by mortality or changes like deformities, haemorrhages or pocks or edema of membranes of embryo, besides detecting presence of antigens in the embryonic fluids by haemagglutination or complement fixation or florescent tests.

4.III.2. Identification

The identification of viruses involve various techniques like recognition of virus growth in cell cultures, electron microscopy, serological and immunological diagnostic techniques.

4.III.2.a. Recognition of Virus Growth in Cell Cultures

Cytopathic Effect

Culture of viruses in living cells do produce specific effects in the cells in which they proliferate and is called cytopathic effect (CPE). Demonstration of CPE helps in identification of viruses. The majority of viruses produce degenerative changes which can be recognized in unstained preparations. These changes are rounding, retraction, syncytium formation and detachment from the surfaces.

Immunofluorescence or Immunoperoxidase

Specific antisera labeled with fluorescent dye or enzyme peroxidase can be used in direct or indirect tests to detect the presence of cytopathic or non-cytopathic viruses in cell cultures.

Haemadsorption

The cultured cells acquire the ability to adsorb the erythrocytes when infected with certain viruses like orthomyxovirus, paramyxovirus or togavirus. This ability of adsorption is due to incorporation of newly synthesized viral protein, responsible for red cell binding, into plasma membrane of cells.

Haemagglutination

The medium of cell cultures infected with some viruses of group myxo or paramyxoviruses acquire the property to clump the erythrocytes of certain species of birds and animals.

Interference

The propagation of one virus in cell cultures usually inhibits the replication of second virus.

Inclusion Body Demonstration

Fixation and staining of cell monolayer can be helpful in the demonstration of virus multipli-cation specific structures (inclusion bodies). The demonstration of inclusion bodies is a valuable diagnostic aid. They may be demonstrated in the cytoplasm e.g. Negri bodies of rabies or in nucleus e.g. chicken pox, Herpes, yellow fever etc.

4.III.2.b. Electron–microscopy

Shape and size of viruses can be determined by electron microscopy. Viruses differ in shape, some are brick like (vaccine virus), filamentous or spherical (influenza virus) or sperm like (bacteriophages). It is a simple, quick and reliable diagnostic method that is being employed in the samples like vesicle fluid, solid warty tissue, faecal samples and serum for the demonstration of viruses. However, it involves expensive equipment and experienced operator. Since viruses have a distinctive morphology of which symmetry is usually a feature that makes it very simple to distinguish them from cellular background. The principle on which this technique is based is that the electron beam cannot penetrate the heavy metal stain but can pass through organic material present, which appears light against dark background. Here in this method a virus containing suspension is mixed with an electron dense stain, usually phosphotungstic acid (30-40g/lit, pH-6) a drop of this mixture is allowed to dry on a grid and examined directly in an electron microscope.

4.III.2.c. Serological Tests

The serological tests are of paramount importance in the diagnosis of viral diseases and have thus been described in detail in Chapter 6.

SECTION-IV

4.IV.1. Isolation and Identification of Parasites

Faecal examination for identification of helminth infestation

Examination of faeces gives an accurate indication and identification of parasites found in alimentary canal and releasing their eggs through feaces. Some times the parasites of respiratory tract can also be diagnosed by faecal examination as the patients oftenly swallow the sputum containing eggs.

Faeces are best collected from rectum as it avoids the danger of contamination. When blood or mucus is present, it should be separated for immediate examination.

4.IV.1.a. Direct Method

It is most simple method that involves following procedure.

1. Small quantity of fecal sample is mixed with sufficient quantity of water on the slide.
2. Cover slip is put over and examined under microscope.
3. Direct microscopical examination of faeces or gut contents is often of value, particularly if there is swarming infection.
4. Motile organisms can be protected from distortion by supporting the cover slip or by the use of hanging drop in a cavity slide.

4.IV.1.b. Sedimentation Method

Preliminary screening of the material followed by flotation and or sedimentation can be used for concentration and separation of parasites or eggs from the bulk of sample material. For easy identification of protozoa eosin stain is used to colours the feacal debris as intense red where-as freshly passed protozoa, including cysts, resist the stain and are thus easily identified as white bodies, even with low power objective. Sedimentation method involves the following procedure:

1. 2 gms of feces are mixed with10 volumes of water and then strained through cloth or coffee strainer.
2. Material is centrifuged at 1000 rpm for 1–2 minutes.

3. Supernatant fluid is discarded and water is added and again centrifuged at 1000rpm for 2 minutes.
4. Supernatant is discarded and sediment is taken on a slide and covered with cover slip.
5. Examination of material is carried under microscope.
6. Samples containing excess of fatty material is treated with ether prior to centrifugation.
7. Parasites of high specific gravity are detected in this method and is best for evaluation of trematode eggs which are of high specific gravity.

4.IV.1.c. Floatation Method

The principle of this method is to bring specific gravity of the fluid to a point at which it is less than that of the particles of the debris but greater than that of the material wished to be collected.

1. 2–5 gms of feces are mixed with water, sieved and centrifuged.
2. Sediment is mixed with sufficient quantity of floatation fluid (saturated solution of sugar, sodium chloride or magnesium sulphate or zinc sulphate).
3. The mixture of sediment and floatation fluid is filled in test tubes up to the top.
4. After 30 minutes of standing or spinning the material, at 1500- 3000 rpm to deposit the debris and bring the ova/protozoa to the surface, a cover slip is placed on the top of the fluid in the test tube.
5. The cover slip is lifted vertically and put on the slide.
6. Examination of slide is carried under 10 to 40x objective of microscope.
7. This procedure is suitable for hook worms, ascaris, trichuris, tape worms, coccidian oocysts and gastro-intestinal parasites of sheep, cattle and horses.

4.IV.2. Cultural Techniques

In cases where eggs in the faecal samples are difficult to diagnose and larvae are readily identified, employment of cultural methods is preferred.

4.IV.2.a. Test Tube Culture

1. Spread a thin (1-2 mm) film of faecse on one side of the middle third of 13x120 mm filter paper strip.
2. Place it in a 15ml centrifuge tube containing 3ml of distilled water with clean side pressed against the side of the tube and bottom end of the strip in water.
3. Store the culture tube in dark at room temperature (24-28°C) for 7 to 10 days.
4. Add water daily to the tube to keep water level above bottom end of paper strip so as to keep faces moist.
5. On reaching infective stage larvae migrate down ward against upward flow of water and when they reach the water level, they sink to the bottom of the tube.
6. The larvae can be seen by using hand lens or pipetted out and examined under microscope.

4.IV.2.b. Charcoal Culture:

1. Mix 1part of soft or softened faeces with 5-10 parts of fine, granular animal charcoal.
2. Dampen it throughout and pack it in a covered but not air tight container.
3. Store the culture container in dark at room temperature (24-28°C) for 7 to 10 days.
4. On reaching infective stage of development, larvae migrate to the surface.
5. A thick pad of soft cotton, cloth or absorbent gauze of appropriate size to fit the culture container, is soaked in warm water and pressed to the culture surface and cover replaced.
6. After half an hour the pad is picked up at the center with forceps and transferred up side down to a sedimentation flask, filled with warm water.
7. Larvae promptly fall into the bottom ot tlask where from they can be pipetted out and examined under microscope.

4.IV.2.c. Culture of Protozoa

Protozoa can be maintained in artificial medium, however, maintenance of fully virulent strains require the use of experimental animals along with passage in usual vector.

Trypanosomes can often be established in blood agar and good growth can be obtained at 25-30°C, but do not retain infectivity. Cultivation can be carried out in 6 -7 days live chick-embryos and infection noticed in 48-72 hours. Tryps have been cultured in Trypticase Soy broth, Blood lysate medium or Novy-Mac Neal-Nicolles medium.

Tryps can be maintained by inoculating mice, rats, rabbits, monkeys and puppies either by depositing the droppings of infected bugs on to mucous membrane or by injecting intraperitoneally the blood from an infected mammalian host. Daily examination of infected animals is carried out for appearance of organism in peripheral blood. Once in peripheral circulation, sub-inoculation should be done.

Babesia, anaplasma and plasmodium have not been cultured successfully, however, can be maintained in their natural, intermediate or definitive hosts. Ticks remain infected for several generations. Anaplasma can be maintained in defibrinated blood for about 3 weeks. Theilaria can be maintained for several days in tissue culture.

Entamoeba can be cultured in Dobell's medium and Trichomonas in Bacto-tryptose broth with 2% dextrose.

Toxoplasma is readily maintained in laboratory animals like mice, rats, hamsters, rabbits, guinea pigs, pigeons or chick embryos and also in tissue cultures.

4.IV.3. Staining Techniques Used in Identification of Blood Parasites

Wright's staining:

Primarily used to stain blood smears, however, has certain bacteriological application in study of phagocytes.

Procedure

1. Fix and stain dry unfixed smears by the Wright's stain that contains methyl alcohol as a fixative.

2. Cover the smear with undiluted stain and allow it to stand for a minute.
3. Dilute the stain on the slide by adding equal volume of phosphate buffer or distilled water and mix it with the help of a pipette by sucking and releasing the fluid in the pipette.
4. Allow the diluted stain to remain on slide for 5 to 10 minutes.
5. Wash the slide by flooding it with same buffer or distilled water.
6. Dry the slide by blotting or in air.

Leishman's Staining

This method of staining is preferably used in staining of blood films for the demonstration of blood parasites.

Procedure

1. Fix and stain dry unfixed smears by Leishman's stain that contains methyl alcohol as a fixative.
2. Cover the smear with undiluted stain and allow it to stand for a minute.
3. Dilute the stain on the slide by adding equal volume of phosphate buffer or distilled water and mix it with the help of a pipette by sucking and releasing the fluid in the pipette.
4. Allow the diluted stain to remain on slide for 5 to 10 minutes.
5. Wash the slide by flooding it with same buffer or distilled water.
6. Dry the slide by blotting or in air.

Giemsa's Staining

This staining method gives the best results for demonstration of spirochaetes and certain protozoa, besides it is useful in demonstration of rickettsia and virus inclusion bodies.

Procedure

1. Make thin smear of blood or culture to be examined on a slide, dry it in air and fix in absolute methyl alcohol for 15 minutes.
2. Stain the slide in a coplin jar with one part of stain and ten parts of buffer solution pH 7.0 for 1 hour to 3 hours.
3. Wash the slide with buffer and dry in air before examining under oil immersion.

Table 4.1: Helminth Parasites of Ruminants and Their Preferred Site of Infestation.

Site of Infestation	*Parasites*
Eye	Thelazia
Brain	Coenurus
Trachea	Mammomonogamus
Oesophagus	Gongylonema
Lungs	Dictyocaulus, Protostrongylus, Muellerius, Cystocaulus, Hydatid cysts.
Aorta	Onchocerca armillata
Liver	Fasciola, Dicrocoelium, Schistosoma, Hydatid cysts.
Rumen	Paramphistomidae, Gastrothylacidae
Abomasum	Haemonchus, Trichostrongylus, Ostertagia
Small intestine	Strongyloides, Bunostomum, Gaigeria, Nematodirus, Chabertia, Toxocara, Cooperia, Moniezia, Trichostrongylus, Stilasia, Ostertagia, Avitellina.
Large intestine	Oesophagostomum, Trichuris
Mesenteric membranes	Schistosoma
Cervical ligaments	Onchocerca gutturosa
Joints	Onchocerca
Body cavity	Cysticercus tenuicollis, Setaria
Muscles	Onchocerca dukei, cysticercus bovis
Skin	Onchocerca dermata

Table 4.2: Helminth Parasites of Birds and Their Preferred Site of Infestation.

Site of Infestation	*Parasites*
Eye	Oxyspirura
Trachea	Syngamus
Oesophagus and crop	Capillaria
Proventriculus	Tetramers
Gizzard	Synhimantus, Cheilospirura, Streptocara
Intestine	Strongyloides, Hartertia, Allodapa, Heterakis, Ascaridia, Capillaria, Davainea, Raillientina, Hymenolepis, Choanotaenia, Fimbriaria, Amoebotaenia, Brachylaemus, Mediorhynchus

Chapter 5

Animal Diseases and their Diagnostic Tools

The majority of live-stock and poultry diseases are spread through widely distributed pathogenic agents in the nature like bacteria, fungi, viruses etc. However, disease conditions reproduced by certain chemical and physical agents, besides nutritional deficiencies can not be ignored.

The very first instrument in tentative diagnosis of a disease is the changed physical, mental, behavioral and feeding patterns (commonly termed as symptoms) of the animal. To arrive at complete and confirmatory diagnosis of a disease, several diagnostic tools are employed for which various types of inputs/samples are required. With the advancement in the scientific research many new, more reliable and less time taking tests have been evolved for the diagnosis of diseases.

SECTION-I

Laboratory Diagnosis of Different Livestock and Poultry Diseases

This section has been framed up in a tabular form to provide a ready reference of various livestock and poultry diseases with their main symptoms, list of various laboratory tests and materials/ samples required for their diagnosis.

Table 5.1: Laboratory Diagnosis of Bacterial Diseases.

Disease (1)	*Causative Agent* (2)	*Species Affected* (3)	*Symptoms* (4)	*Diagnostic Tests* (5)	*Materials Required* (6)
Actinobacillosis (wooden tongue)	Actinobacillus Lignieresii	Cattle and sheep	Swelling of tongue, salivation nodules and ulcers on the sides of tongue enlargement of sub-maxillary and parotid nodules that often rupture with discharge. In sheep lesions are purulent on facial skin and lips.	Staining of pus smears, isolation and identification of organism by cultural methods.	Pus on swabs or in sterilized vials from excised nodules or abscesses
Actinomycosis (lumpy jaw)	Actinomyces bovis	Cattle, pigs and horses occasionally	Hard, immovable bony swelling followed by granulomatous, suppurative abcesses involving mandible bone or maxilla.	Demonstration of organism in pus smears, crushed sulfur granules. Culture, isolation and identification of organism.	Fresh material from suppurative lesions on swabs or in sterile containers.
Anthrax	Bacillus anthracis	Man and animals	Septicemia, sudden death, oozing of tarry blood from natural orifices, spleenomegaly.	Examination of stained blood smears, isolation & identification of organism, FAT, guinea pig inoculation, Ascoli's test.	Avoid opening of carcass, swabs and smears of peri-pheral blood. Piece of tissue (Ear).

contd...

Table 5.1–Contd...

(1)	(2)	(3)	(4)	(5)	(6)
Bacillary hemoglobinuria. (red water disease)	Clostridium haemolyticum	Cattle and sheep	High fever, hemoglobinuria and icterus, necrotic infarcts in liver. Cessation of feeding, lactation and defecation. Abdominal pain with arched back posture.	Demonstration of organisms in smears from infarcts by staining and FAT test. Isolation and identification by culture	Portions of liver with infarct (fresh and preserved in formalin).
Black quarter	Clostidium chauvoei and Cl. septicum	Cattle and sheep	High fever, lameness, emphysematous gangrene involving thigh muscles. Complete anorexia, ruminal stasis.	Demonstration of organisms in infected muscle smears by FAT and staining. Culture & isolation of organism.	Portions of gangre-nous muscle & affected muscle or fluid smears.
Botulism	Clostridium botulinum	Domestic, wild animals and birds.	Progressive motor paralysis affecting muscles of limbs, jaw and throat. Paralysis starts from hind quarters and progresses to fore-quarters, head and neck.	Mouse inoculation test of blood, liver extract, serum or suspected food. Toxin neutralization tests.	Serum, suspected food, tied off stomach and a portion of small intestine and liver.
Brucellosis *(zoonotic disease)*	Brucella abortus, B.melitensis B. ovis, B. canis, B.suis	Cattle, buffalo,sheep, dog, pig and man.	Abortions in late pregnancy (7-9 months in cattle),metritis, infertility, orchitis, epididymitis, infection of testicles, and accessory sex glands. Similar symptoms in dogs.	Plate or tube agglutination test, ELISA, Brucella ring test, Rose Bengal agglutination test, CFT, isolation of organism by culture or guinea pig inoculation.	Serum, placenta, cotyledons, aborted fetus, vaginal mucus or uterine exudate, milk, semen and testes.

contd...

Table 5.1–Contd...

(1)	(2)	(3)	(4)	(5)	(6)
Bovine mastitis	Streptococcus, Staphylococcus, E.coli, Pseudomonas, Corynebacterium, Actinomyces, Mycoplasma, Nocardia, Candida sp.	Cattle, sheep, goat and pig	Inflammation and edema of mammary gland mainly the milk cistern, abnormalities of milk including discolouration accompanied by clots and flakes, watery milk. Systemic reaction may include fever, depression, anorexia or toxemia.	Isolation and identification of organism by cultural techniques and drug sensitivity. Milk ELISA for Staphy. Mastitis tests like cell counts in milk, Bromothymol blue test, Calfornia mastitis test.	Milk samples (fresh and insterile vials) at refrigeration temperature.
Braxy	Clostridium septicum	Sheep	Abomasitis with toxemia	FAT, isolation and identification of organism	Smears from incised abomasal lesions
Calf diphtheria	Fusobacterium necrophorum	Young calves	Acute toxemia, fever, necrotic ulcers involving the mucous membranes of mouth, larynx or pharynx or may extend to nose, trachea and lungs	Demonstration of organism in smears from lesions, isolation and identification of organism.	Material collected on swabs from the lesions.
Caseous lymphadenitis	Corynebacterium pseudotuberculosis	Sheep	Caseous necrosis and abscessation of precrural and prescapular lymphnodes followed by mediastinal, bronchial & sublumber lymph nodes.	Isolation and identification of the organism by culture.	Fresh pus collected on swabs.

contd...

Table 5.1–Contd...

(1)	(2)	(3)	(4)	(5)	(6)
Chlamydiosis (Enzootic abortion of ewes, sporadic bovine encephalo-myelitis)	Chlamydia psittaci	Domestic animals	Placentitis, abortions, stillbirths, premature lambing, SBE characterized by neurological form with purulent meningitis. There is dypnea, cough, catarrhal nasal discharge, stifnes, staggering, circling.	Examinations of stained smears, FAT, CFT, isolation and identification by culture in chick embryo.	Fresh placenta, fetus, Serum sample. Portions of brain, pericardium, pleura and lung (fresh and fixed)
Colibacillosis	Escherichia coli	Very young calves and pigs	Depression, fever, anorexia, yellow watery diarrhea, dehydration, emaciation and acidosis.	Isolation of organisms and identification of antigens in culture by agglutination, FAT of fecal smears	Portions of small intestine, liver and spleen, fecal swabs.
Contagious Bovine Pleuro-pneumonia	Mycoplasma mycoides	Cattle less frequent in other ruminants	Fibrinous broncho-pneumonia with consolidation of lungs and pleurisy.	CFT, ELISA, AGPT, FAT, isolation and identification of organism and gross pathology.	Serum samples, tissues and fluid from affected lungs.
Enterotoxemia	Clostridium perfringens	Sheep, lambs, calves, piglets & horses.	Diarrhea, dysentery, convulsions, ataxia and coma. Animals often found dead.	Lab. animal inoculation followed by neutralization tests, demonstration and culture of organisms from duodenal mucosa.	20-30 ml ileac contents in tied off intestine, portions of duodenum.

contd...

Table 5.1–Contd...

(1)	*(2)*	*(3)*	*(4)*	*(5)*	*(6)*
Erysipelas	Erysipelothrix rhusiopathiae	Primarily swine, may affect sheep and poultry	Acute septicemia with fever, depression and death. Skin form with fever, raised, red to purple areas turning into scabs. Arthritic form with lameness, periarticular fibrosis of stifle and hock joints. Endocarditis with dyspnea, skin discolouration of extremities, abnormal cardiac sounds	Isolation and identification of organism, demonstration of Gram-positive rods in fresh blood smears and histopathology.	Heart blood, fresh portions of kidney, spleen, liver. Blood smears in acute form, swabs from affected joints and tissues.
Foot rot	Fusobacterium necrophorum	Cattle	Pain, swelling of claws or coronet, lameness and fever.	Diagnosis based on clinical signs. Demonstration of organisms in stained smears.	Smears of pus from the lesions.
Glanders (Farcy)	Pseudomonas mallei	Horses, mules and donkeys.	Septicemia with fever, cough and nasal discharge. Chronic form characterized by nodules eventually ulcerative involving either nasal mucosa or lungs or skin.	Isolation and identification of organism by culture. Mullein test.	Swabs from ulcers or incised nodules, aspirated pus from nodules. Fresh and fixed portions of nodules and affected lung.

contd...

Table 5.1–Contd...

(1)	*(2)*	*(3)*	*(4)*	*(5)*	*(6)*
Hemorrhagic septicemia (HS)	Pasturella multocida	Cattle and buffaloes.	Edematous swelling in the head, throat and brisket region, swollen and hemorrhagic lymph nodes and subserous petechial hemorrhages.	Isolation and identification of organism by culture or lab animal (mice & rabbit) inoculation.	Swabs from heart blood, liver, spleen and lymph nodes and or portions of these tissues.
Infectious Bovine Kerato-conjectivitis	Moraxella bovis	Cattle	Photophobia, lacrimation, conjunctivitis and keratitis, resulting into corneal ulceration and opacity.	Isolation and identification of M. bovis by culture.	Conjectival swabs in transport medium
Infectious Necrotic Hepatitis (Black Disease)	Clostridium novyi {typeB}	Sheep and cattle	Acute, fatal toxicity, Necrosis of liver tissue, black appearance of skin.	Histopathological examination, guinea pig inoculation for isolation of organism and FAT.	Fresh and fixed portions of liver, smears of necrotic liver lesions.
Leptospirosis	Leptospira interrogans, L. canicola, L.icterohaemo-rrhagiae, L. pomona	Domestic animals, horses, dogs, pigs	Abortions (in late pregnancy in bovines), infertility, fever, interstitial nephritis, depression, capillary damage, petecheal hemorrhages in mucosae, hemoglobinuria, icterus.	Silver impregnation staining of kidney smears, Demonstration of leptospira in urine by dark field examination, isolation and identification by culture, plate agglutination, FAT of kidney and urine and histopathology.	Serum samples, urine samples, portions of kidney and liver (fresh and fixed) and fetal tissue. Formalin added urine (7.5% of 10% formalin)

contd...

Table 5.1–Contd...

(1)	*(2)*	*(3)*	*(4)*	*(5)*	*(6)*
Listeriosis	Listeria monocytogens	Cattle, sheep, goat, horse, swine and birds.	Important cause of abortions, kerato-conjectivitis and ophthalmitis in sheep and cattle. In nervous form of the disease there is circling with a history of feeding silage.	Tube agglutination test, isolation and identification of organism, histopathology of micro-abscesses in the brain stem.	Serum samples, portions of liver, fetus, placenta (fresh and fixed).
Malignant edema	Clostidium septicum	Cattle, sheep, goat, pigs and horses.	Gangrenous process begins in skeletal muscles becoming red, gelatinous, with little gas and pits on pressure.	FAT of smears, culture of the organism may also be attempted.	Aspirated material from the lesions for smears and culture or portions of affected muscle
Paratuberculosis (Johne's Disease)	Mycobacte-rium paratuber-culosis	Cattle, sheep and goats.	Emaciation with recurrent fetid diarrhea.	Isolation and identification of organism, examination of smears for acid-fast bacteria, Johnin test, CFT, immuno-diffusion test and ELISA.	Fecal sample from the rectum, tissue from ileocecal junction and adjacent lymph-nodes,smears from pinched mucosa of the rectal wall or from mesenteric nodes. Serum samples.

contd...

Table 5.1–Contd...

(1)	*(2)*	*(3)*	*(4)*	*(5)*	*(6)*
Q fever	Coxiella burnetii	Cattle, sheep, goat and man.	Anorexia, abortions in goats 2-4 weeks before term.	FAT, CFT and agglutination tests.	Serum samples, milk sample, fetus and placenta.
Salmonellosis	Salmorella species	Domestic animals, lab. animals and birds	Young animals develop septicemia where as adult animals show chronic or acute enteritis. Fever, diarrhea and colic.	Isolation and identification of organism, AGPT, Tube agglutination test and histopathology.	Rectal swabs, fresh and fixed portions of intestine, liver, spleen, lymph nodes. Serum samples
Strangles	Streptococcus ecui	Young equines	Rhinitis, pharyngitis followed by abscesses in inter-mandibular and para-pharyngeal lymph nodes.	Isolation and identification of organism by culture.	Fresh pus on swab from an excised abscess.
Tetanus	Clostridium tetani	Farm animals, most commonly in horse and sheep.	Gradual onset of stiffness, hyperesthesia, titanic spasms of all voluntary muscles (wooden horse appearance)	Isolation and identification of organism. Clinical findings& observation of organism in stained smears from a wound.	Pus or necrosed tissue from wound in anaerobic transport media.

contd...

Table 5.1–Contd...

(1)	(2)	(3)	(4)	(5)	(6)
Tuberculosis	Mycobacterium bovis	Cattle, other domestic animals and poultry	Formation of granulomatous nodules (tubercles) in lungs, associated lymph nodes and mesenteric lymph nodes.	Demonstration of acid-fast organisms in the smears from lesions. Tuberculin test, ELISA, PCR, radiography.	Serum samples, fresh and fixed portions of lungs, intestinal lymph nodes and tubercular tissue.
Ulcerative lymphangitis	Corynebacterium pseudo-tuberculosis	Horses and mules	Ulcerative nodules in skin, lymph vessels and nodes in the region of fetlock. Inflammation of lymphatics without abscessation.	Isolation and identification of organism.	Pus collected on swab from excised nodule.

Table 5.2: Laboratory Diagnosis of Fungal Diseases.

Disease (1)	*Causative Agent* (2)	*Species Affected* (3)	*Symptoms* (4)	*Diagnostic Tests* (5)	*Materials Required* (6)
Aspergillosis	Aspergillus fumigatus	Animals and birds	Abortions in cattle, granulomatous, necrotized lesions in lungs. Brooder's pneumonia in birds with loss of appetite, polypnea, fever and listlessness.	Wet mount examination, culture of the organism, agar gel immunodiffusion tests and histopathology.	Swabs of nasal cavity, fresh and fixed curetted material from lesions, trans-thoracic biopsy, serum samples.
Blastomycosis	Blastomyces dermatitidis	Dog and man, rarely other animals	Granulomatous, suppurative nodules in lungs with frequent metastasis to skin, bone and other tissues.	Demonstration of single budding yeasts in gram staining smears, infected tissues and exudates. Isolation by culture. CFT & immunodiffusion tests.	Transthoracic biopsy, transtracheal aspirations and granulomatous nodules or abscesses and serum samples.
Candidiasis	Candida albicans	Domestic animals and pets	Infection of mucous membranes of alimentary tract, genital tract and infrequently of lungs, heart and kidneys.	Demonstration of organism in smears and wet mounts, isolation by culture, histopathology of tissues & immunodiffusion tests.	Material collected from deeper layers of affected tissue (fresh and fixed). Serum samples.

contd...

Table 5.2–Contd...

(1)	*(2)*	*(3)*	*(4)*	*(5)*	*(6)*
Cryptococcosis	Cryptoco-ccus neoformans	Cattle, sheep, goat, horses, dogs, cats.	Manifested as a paranasal infection that often extends to meninges, brain and lungs. granulomatous lesions are characteri-stics.	Demonstration of organisms in wet mounts or stained smears of material taken from lesions.	Material from nasal passages or from granulomatous lesions. Biopsies and or CSF collected. Portions of affected tissues fresh and fixed.
Dermatophy-tosis (ring worm)	Microsporum & Trichophyton species	Domestic and other animals.	Infects keratin containing tissues like skin, nails and hair. Lesions spread out from a central locus forming circular, patchy lesions	Examination of wet mounts for spores and fungal elements, culture, isolation and identification	Skin scrapings from edges of lesion, plucked hairs.
Histoplasm-osis	Histoplasma capsulatum	Domestic animals and humans	Infection of reticulo-endothelial system. Granulomas of lymph nodes, internal organs like lungs and intestinal tract.	Demonstration of yeast cells in stained smears, culture and histopathology. CFT and immunodiffusion tests.	Excised lymph nodes, lymphnode or liver biopsies, fresh and fixed portions of lung, liver, spleen, intestinal wall or skin with granulomas. Serum samples.

contd...

Table 5.2–Contd...

(1)	*(2)*	*(3)*	*(4)*	*(5)*	*(6)*
Sporotrichosis	Sporothrix schenckii	Horses, mules, dogs, cats and pigs.	Suppurative nodules of skin, subcutis, superficial lymphatics and lymph nodes.	FAT, examination of stained or wet mount smears and culture and identification of organism.	Pus from the excised lesions
Zygomycosis/ Mucormycosis	Mucor/ Rhizopus/ Mortierella species	Cattle, horse, pigs, dogs, cats and other animals	Focal granulomatous lesions in lymph nodes of lungs or intestinal tract. Sometimes associated with ulcerations of rumen, abomasums or stomach of cattle and pigs.	Demonstration of fungal elements in wet mounts or in stained tissue sections	Fresh and fixed portions of lymph nodes with lesion

Table 5.3: Laboratory Diagnosis of Viral Diseases.

Disease (1)	*Causative Agent* (2)	*Species Affected* (3)	*Symptoms* (4)	*Diagnostic Tests* (5)	*Materials Required* (6)
African Horse Sickness	Orbivirus	Equines	Pulmonary form with fever, cough, choking and frothy fluid from nostrils. Cardiac form with swelling of head, neck, eyelids, brisket, thorax and abdomen.	Virus isolation in mouse or horse, CFT, ELISA, Virus neutralization and immunodiffusion tests.	Unclotted blood, clotted blood 5-6 days after highest temperature and portions of spleen, heart, lung, liver and kidney.
Blue tongue	Orbovirus	Cattle, sheep, goat and wild ruminants	Fever, leucopenia, erosive inflammation of mouth, tongue and lips. Nasal and ocular discharge. Stiffness, laminitis, coronitis.	CFT, AGPT, Immuno-diffusion test, FAT, Virus neutralization, ELISA, radio-immunoassay. Virus isolation by intravenous chick embryo inoculation.	Serum samples, whole blood, specimens of spleen, mesenteric nodes and aborted fetuses.
Bovine leucosis (malignant lymphoma)	Retro virus {oncorna group}	Cattle	Fatal, malignant neoplasia of reticuloendothelial system. Development of tumor growth in many organs, enlargement of superficial lymph nodes.	Agar gel immunodiffusion test, RIA, histopathological study of affected tissues. Isolation of virus using tissue culture on lamb spleen cells.	Serum samples, affected tissue (fresh and fixed), uncoagulated blood.

contd...

Table 5.3–Contd...

(1)	(2)	(3)	(4)	(5)	(6)
Bovine Spongiform Encephalo-pathy (BSE/ Mad cow disease)	Prion	Cattle	Degenerative changes in central nervous system. Loss of weight and condition, aggression, gait ataxia, tremors, excitability and generalized paresis and death.	Histopathological findings of neuronal, vaculation, gliosis and neuronal loss. Mice inoculation with fresh brain and cord.	Fresh and fixed portions of brain and cord.
Bovine Virus Diarrhoea (BVD)	Toga virus	Cattle	Inflammation and erosions of mucous membrane of alimentary tract with diarrhea, abortions.	Virus isolation and identification, FAT, virus neutralization and histopathology.	Swabs of nasal discharge, feces, Fresh & fixed portions of spleen, intestine, lympnodes, fetal liver & kidney. Blood, blood smears, serum.
Canine distemper	Paramyxo Virus	Dogs	Diphasic fever, leukopenia, coryza followed by bronchitis, catarrhal pneumonia, gastroenteritis and neurological signs.	FAT, histopathology of lung, stomach, pancreas for inclusion bodies, microscopic evaluation of demyelination with inclusions in glial cells, ELISA and virus isolation.	Conjunctival, tracheal, vaginal scrapings in live animals. Fresh and fixed portions of intestine, pancreas, stomach, lung and brain. Serum samples.

contd...

Table 5.3–Contd...

(1)	*(2)*	*(3)*	*(4)*	*(5)*	*(6)*
Contagious ecthyma (*zoonotic, ORF*)	Parapox virus	Sheep and Goat	Formation of papules, vesicles, pustules and scabs on lips, mucous membranes of oral cavity, nostrils.	Demonstration of parapox virus in smears or sections of biopsies or in homogenates by electron microscope.	Scrapings and biopsies from the lesions.
Cow pox (*zoonotic*)	Orthopox virus	Bovines	Formation of papules, vesicles on teats and udder, loss of milk production.	Isolation in cell cultures or chick embryo. Examination of vesicular fluid by electron microscope.	Vesicular fluid and tissues from the lesions.
Ephemeral fever	Rhabdo virus	Cattle and Buffaloes	Fever, lameness, stiffness, muscular tremors, enlargement of superficial lymph nodes, short course with spontaneous recovery.	Virus isolation in mice and hamsters and identification by neutralization tests.	Unclotted blood to be taken at acute phase of disease.
Equine infectious anemia (swamp fever)	Retrovirus	Equines	Intermittent fever, loss of condition, anemia, icterus, edema, petechial hemorrhages.	Agar gel immunodiffusion, c-ELISA,	Serum samples

contd...

Table 5.3–Contd...

(1)	(2)	(3)	(4)	(5)	(6)
Equine influenza	Orthomyxo virus {type-A influenza virus}	Equines	Highly contagious respiratory disease, with dry, hacking cough.	HI test, CFT, Virus neutralization. Isolation and identification in chick embryos or cell cultures.	Serum samples, nasal swabs and tracheal wash.
Foot and mouth disease (FMD)	Picorna virus	Cloven footed animals	Vesicular formation followed by erosions of the epithelium of mouth, nares, muzzle, feet, udder and teats. Reduced milk yield, lameness, mastitis and sometimes abortion.	CFT, AGID, ELISA, FAT, virus isolation in cell cultures and identification by neutralization tests.	Vesicle fluid, epithelial flaps from lesions of tongue and gums in tissue culture medium containing antibiotics or 50% phosphate buffer glycerin saline. Serum samples
Hog Cholera	Togavirus	Pigs	Acute form with viremia, high grade fever and mortality. Chronic form results in congenital defects in fetus.	FAT, AGPT with known immune sera using pancreas as source antigen. Indirect enzyme labeled antibody test.	Blood samples, fixed sections of intestine & brain. Fresh portions of pancreas, lymph node, tonsil and spleen.
Infectious Canine Hepatitis	Canine Adenovirus type 1	Dogs	Anorexia, intense thirst, fever, tonsillitis, conjectivitis, edema of head, neck and lower abdomen, epistaxis, vomiting, diarrhea and pain. Nervous symptoms like depression, dis-orientation and seizures.	FAT of liver biopsies and cell cultures. Isolation in cell cultures. Virus neutralization test. Histo-pathological examination for inclusion bodies.	Liver biopsies, urine and nasal swabs, serum samples, fresh and fixed portions of liver, spleen and gall bladder.

Table 5.3–Contd...

(1)	*(2)*	*(3)*	*(4)*	*(5)*	*(6)*
Infectious bovine rhinotracheitis (IBR)	Bovine Herpes-virus 1.	Cattle	Respiratory infection with nasal and ocular discharge, dispnea, edema, hemorrhages and necrosis of mucosa of upper respiratory tract in acute cases. Encephalitis in 2-3 months old calves, enteritis in young calves, pustular vulvo-vaginitis and balanoposthitis and abortions.	Virus neutralization tests, ELISA, FAT of tissue sections and isolation and identification in cell cultures.	Nasal, vaginal and preputial swabs, fresh and fixed tissues from affected organs. Fetal liver, kidney and lung. Serum samples (acute and convalescent).
Malignant Catarrhal Fever	Herpes-virus	Cattle and buffaloes	Catarrhal and mucopurulent inflammation of mucous membranes. The head and eye form of the disease is most common with erosions of oral and nasal mucosa , severe kerato-conjectivitis, muco-purulant discharge, high fever, severe diarrhea, convulsions and tremors.	Diagnosis based on clinical signs and histopathological findings of vasculitis, lymphocytic infiltration and proliferation in most organs. Rabbit inoculation results in nervous symptoms. Virus isolation and PCR	Fresh leukocytes, spleen, lymph nodes, tonsils, thyroids and adrenals. Fixed portions from liver, spleen, lymph nodes and lesions of alimentary tract. Serum samples.

contd...

Table 5.3–Contd...

(1)	*(2)*	*(3)*	*(4)*	*(5)*	*(6)*
Papillomatosis	Papillomaviruses	Cattle, goat, horse and dogs.	Formation of benign tumors (cauliflower like in cattle) involving skin, oral and even genital mucosa. Elevated tumors in dogs.	Clinical diagnosis on the basis of characteristic lesions and histopathology of lesions.	Biopsies from the lesions.
Peste Des Petits Ruminants (PPR)	Morbilivirus	Sheep and goat	Closely related to RP. Fever, nasal discharge, oral mucosal erosions, diarrhea and emaciation. Marked leucopenia with neutrophilia.	Isolation and identification of virus. CFT, serum neutralization test, agar gel diffusion test with lymph node as source of antigen and hematology.	Serum samples, lymph node biopsy, uncoagulated blood
Progressive Pneumonia (Maedi – Visna)	Retrovirus	Sheep and goat.	Chronic course with signs of dyspnea, circling, trembling, deviation of head, emaciation, progressive paresis.	CFT, virus neutralization, isolation and identification in cell cultures, histopathology of lungs and brain.	Serum samples, fresh and fixed portions of lung, cerebrum and cerebellum.
Pseudocow pox (Milker's Nodules)	Parapox virus	Cattle	Small papules on the udder and teats, turning to vesicles or pustules and finally scabs. The infection may spread as purplish nodules on fingers and hands.	Electron microscopy of vesicular fluid, culture and identification in cell cultures.	Fluid from the vesicles under refrigeration. Scabs and scrapings from lesions.

contd...

Table 5.3–Contd...

(1)	(2)	(3)	(4)	(5)	(6)
Pseudorabies (Aujeszky's Disease)	Herpesvirus	Swine, rodents farm animals, Dogs and cats	Incoordination, paddling movements and convulsions in young pigs. Intense pruritis and encephalitis in other animals.	FAT, virus neutralization, ELISA, virus isolation and identification and demonstration of inclusion bodies by histopathology	Fresh and fixed portions of brain, skin and sub-cutaneous tissue from the site of pruritis. Serum samples.
Rabies	Rhabdovirus	Warm blooded mammals	Animals show changes in behaviour with anxiety, apprehension. Aimless wandering, excitement, irritability, biting attempts, altered barking, muscle paralysis, salivation, convulsion, ataxia, paralysis and death.	FAT of smears from hippo-campus and salivary glands, demonstration of negri bodies in the neurons of hippocampus.	Entire carcass and head.
Rift Valley Fever	Bunyavirus	Cattle, sheep, goats and man.	Fever, hepatic necrosis with high mortality in young and abortions in pregnant animals.	Isolation and identification of virus. Serum neutralization, CFT, FAT and even transmission tests to mice and sheep.	Serum samples, fresh and fixed portions of liver, liver impression smears. Aborted fetuses.

contd...

Table 5.3–Contd...

(1)	*(2)*	*(3)*	*(4)*	*(5)*	*(6)*
Rinderpest (RP)	Morbilivirus	Cattle, sheep, goat, swine	Highly contagious,febrile disease with severe congestion, hemorrhages and erosions of mucous membranes of alimentary tract and diarrhea.	Virus isolation in tissue culture, CFT, immuno-diffusion, ELISA, histo-pathology and virus-neutralization. A cross protection test using immune and susceptible cattle.	Heparinized blood, mesenteric lymph nodes and spleen in acute phase in frozen state. Fixed portions of tonsil, liver, spleen, kidney and intestines with lesions. Serum samples,
Rotavirus infection (calf scours)	Rotavirus	Calves, foals, lambs and piglets.	Disease of young ones with enteritis, profuse watery diarrhea of sudden onset and dehydration	FAT of fecal and intestinal smears, ELISA, RNA-PAGE, agglutination test and demons-tration of virus in the fecal sample by electron microscope	Fresh and fixed portions of ileum and jejunum. Feces in transport medium shortly after onset of disease.
Scrapie	Prion	Sheep and goats	Degenerative disease of nervous system with signs of incessant itching, depression, muscular tremor, ataxia, in-coordination, excitability and death.	Mice or sheep inoculation and histopathology of brain tissue showing vacuolation of neurons.	Fresh and fixed portions of brain and spinal cord.

contd...

Table 5.3–Contd...

(1)	*(2)*	*(3)*	*(4)*	*(5)*	*(6)*
Sheep and Goat Pox	Poxvirus	Sheep and goat	Fever, pox lesions (papules, pustules and scabs) on unwooled skin, buccal, digestive and respiratory tract mucosa.	Demonstration of pox virus in tissue smears or sections with, electron microscope and FAT.CFT, agar gel immuno-diffusion and virus neutralization. Isolation of virus in cell cultures or chick embryo.	Vesicular fluid and tissues from the lesions.
Vesicular Exanthema of swine	Calcivirus	Pigs	Formation of vesicles on feet, snout, lips and mouth with erosions.	CFT, AGID, ELISA, FAT, virus isolation in cell cultures and identification by neutralization tests.	Vesicle fluid, epithelial flaps in tissue culture medium containing antibiotics or buffered glycerin saline. Serum samples.
Vesicular Stomatitis	Rhabdovirus	Cattle, horses and pigs	Vesicle formation followed by erosions in oral mucous membrane and skin of feet.	CFT. Virus neutralization, isolation of virus from the lesions.	Epithelial tissue covering the vesicles in buffered glycerol or frozen. Vesicular fluid, saliva.

Table 5.4: Laboratory Diagnosis of Parasitic Diseases.

Disease (1)	*Causative Agent* (2)	*Species Affected* (3)	*Symptoms* (4)	*Diagnostic Tests* (5)	*Materials Required* (6)
Amphistomiasis	Paramphistomum Cervi, P. microbothrioides P. liorchis	Cattle and sheep	Fetid diarrhea, weakness, dehydration, anorexia, sub-maxillary edema, pallor and rough coat	Examination of flukes in dung. Clinical findings correlated to environmental conditions and presence of snails.	Dung samples
Ascariasis	Toxacara vitulorum, Ascaris suum, A. Lumbricoide Parascaris equorum	Cattle, sheep, pig and horse	Poor growth, diarrhea and colic. Acute hepatitis or respiratory distress as a result of migration of immature worms.	Examination of eggs in feces. Serum transaminase detection which is elevated.	Fecal and serum samples.
Bunostomiasis	Bunostomum phlebotomum, Bunostomum trigonocephalum	Cattle, sheep and pigs	Stamping and licking of feet, constipation and colic followed by diarrhea, anemia, pallor, anasarca.	Identification of eggs in feces and or larvae at culture of feces.	Fecal samples.
Hemonchosis	Hemonchus contortus	Sheep, goat cattle	Lethargy, muscular weakness, pallor, anasarca under lower jaw and ventral abdomen. Hemorrhagic gastritis, dark coloured feces in acute cases.	Examination of fecal sample for presence of eggs and identification of larvae in fecal culture.	Fecal samples.

contd...

Table 5.4–Contd...

(1)	(2)	(3)	(4)	(5)	(6)
Hepatic fascioliasis	Fasciola hepatica F. gigantica	Domestic animals	Submandibular edema, anemia, pallor, chronic diarrhea, loss of weight and fall in production.	Identification of eggs in feces, ELISA and presence of large flukes in bile ducts and liver.	Fecal sample, portions of liver (fresh and fixed) serum samples.
Lung worm infestation (verminous pneumonia)	Dictyocaulus viviparous. D. fileria. D.arnfieldi. Metastongylus apri	Cattle, sheep, horse and pig	Disease of young animals. Fever, pneumonia, bronchial cough with nasal discharge, tachycardia, dyspnea, polypnea and even consolidation.	Examination of larvae in feces, CFT, Intradermal sensitivity test	Fecal sample, serum samples.
Strongylosis (red worm infestation)	Strongylus vulgaris	Horses	Poor growth, weakness, loss of condition, anorxia, dull, diarrhea and intermittent colic.	Identification of eggs in feces, detection of betaglobulins which gets increased and palpation of cranial mesenteric artery per rectum which becomes thickened.	Fecal and serum samples.
Strongyloidosis	Strongyloides papillosus. S. westerni. S. ransonmi	Farm animals	Anorexia, loss of weight, catarrhal enteritis, diarrhea and anemia. Dermatitis on skin penetration.	Identification of eggs in feces.	Fecal sample.

contd...

Table 5.4–Contd...

(1)	*(2)*	*(3)*	*(4)*	*(5)*	*(6)*
Tapeworm infestation	Moniezia expansa. M. benedini. Helictomera giardi.	Young farm animals	Unthriftiness, poor coat, vague digestive disturbances, constipation, diarrhea, dysentery and anemia. Stunting and pot belly.	Demonstration of segments of tapeworm in feces and identification of embryonated eggs in feces.	Fecal samples.
Trichuriasis (whip worm)	Trichuri ovis T. discolor T. globulosa T. suis	Cattle, sheep, goat, pig	Anorexia, weight loss, diarrhea with mucus and blood.	Demonstration of characteristic yellow barrel shaped eggs in the feces.	Fecal sample.

Table 5.5: Laboratory Diagnosis of Protozoal Diseases.

Disease (1)	*Causative Agent* (2)	*Species Affected* (3)	*Symptoms* (4)	*Diagnostic Tests* (5)	*Materials Required* (6)
Anaplasmosis	Anaplasma marginale, A. ovis	Cattle and other ruminants	Fever, anorexia, anemia and icterus, debility and emaciation. Enlarged and edematous lymph glands. No hemoglobinuria.	Blood smear examination, rapid card agglutination, FAT, CFT	Uncoagulated / whole blood, serum/ plasma.
Babesiosis	Babesisa, Bovis, B. bigemina, B. major, B. ovis, B. equi, B. caballi	Cattle, sheep, goat, pigs and horses	Fever, anorexia, depression, intra-vascular hemolysis, anemia, hemoglobinuria, significant pallor. In horses edema of fetlocks or abdomen and colic.	Demonstration of parasite in peripheral blood film. CFT, FAT, Agglutination test, ELISA, hematology	Peripheral blood smears, un-coagulated blood, paired serum samples
Coccidiosis	Eimeria spps. E. zuernii, E. bovis, E. arloingi	Young cattle, sheep, goat, pig, horse and donkey	Hemorrhagic enteritis, severe diarrhea with foul smell, streaks or clots of blood, straining and anemia. Nervous signs in calves in acute coccidiosis.	Demonstration of oocytes in feces or schizonts and oocytes in scrapings of mucosa.	Fecal sample and or fresh and fixed intestinal loops.

contd...

Table 5.5–Contd...

(1)	*(2)*	*(3)*	*(4)*	*(5)*	*(6)*
Theilariasis	Theilaria annulata, T. parva, T. mutans, T. bovis, T. ovis	Cattle	Fever, hypertrophy of lymph glands, leucopenia, kidney infarcts, lung edema.	Ring, oval, rod or comma shaped bodies in RBCs. Demonstration of Koch's blue bodies in cytoplasm of leucocytes, in lymph gland or spleen juice. Culture in rodent spleen tissue.	Uncoagulated blood. Fresh portions of lymph glands and spleen or biopsy of lymph glands.
Trichomoniasis	Trichomonas fetus	Cattle	Infertility, abortions (2-4 months), pyometra and repeat breeding. Swelling of prepuce and pain in bull.	Cervical mucus agglutination test, hanging drop examination of fetal stomach and uterine exudates. Culture in kidney tissue monolyers.	Uterine or cervical mucus, washings of fetal stomach, amniotic and allantoic fluids. Preputial washing in bull.
Toxoplasmosis (*zoonotic*)	Toxoplasma gondii	Animals and man	Emaciation, enlargement of lymph-nodes, fever, encephalitis, pneumonitis, enterocolitis, abortions and stillbirths.	Demonstration of parasite in spinal fluid, CFT, Sabin-Feldman dye test, FAT and histopathology. Inoculation in lab. animals, chick embryo.	Spinal fluid, Serum samples, fresh and fixed portions of brain, lymph nodes, liver, spleen.

contd...

Table 5.5–Contd...

(1)	*(2)*	*(3)*	*(4)*	*(5)*	*(6)*
Trypanosomiasis	Trypanosoma vivex, Tr. congolense. Tr. Evansi	Cattle, buffalo, sheep, goat, camel and horses	Fever, emaciation, anemia, spleenomegaly, enlargement of lymph nodes, hemorrhages on mucosal and serosal surfaces.	Demonstration of parasite in peripheral blood smears, lymph node smears, plasma after centrifugation of blood, CFT and animal inoculation (sheep, goat, rodents).	Blood and lymph node smears, Uncoagulated blood, serum samples,
Dourine	Trypanosoma equiperdum	Horse	Inflammation of external genetalia, paraphimosis, enlargement of inguinal lymph nodes, mucopurulent urethral discharge or ulcerations of vaginal mucosa.	Demonstration of parasite in discharges, vaginal and urethral washings. CFT and dourine test.	Preputial or vaginal washings, serum samples.

Table 5.6: Laboratory Diagnosis of Metabolic Diseases.

Disease (1)	*Causative Agent (2)*	*Species Affected (3)*	*Symptoms (4)*	*Diagnostic Tests (5)*	*Materials Required (6)*
Downer's Cow Syndrome	Traumatic injury to muscles and nerves or recumbency as a complications of hypocal-cemic parturient paresis.	Cattle, Sheep, Goat	Animal is unable to rise or makes no efforts, after treatment for parturient paresis but is bright, alert, eats & drinks well. Tachycardia, arrhythmia in some.	Clinical manifestations, Serum biochemistry reveals hypo-calcemia, hypo-phosphatemia, ketonuria and elevated SGOT & CPK	Serum samples or uncoagulated blood under refrigeration.
Ketosis (Pregnancy Toxemia)	Hypoglycemia/ negative energy balance	Cattle, sheep, goat	Loss of body weight, cutaneous elasticity and sub-cutaneous fat. Fall in yield and appetite. Characteristic odour of ketones in breath, milk and urine. Nervous signs may begin quite suddenly that include straddling, crossing of legs, circling movements, apparent blindness, hyper - aesthesia.	Clinical findings and serum biochemistry revealing, hypoglycemia, ketonemia, elevated free fatty acids and ketonuria.	Serum samples, uncoagulated blood and urine sample under refrigeration.

contd...

Table 5.6–Contd...

(1)	*(2)*	*(3)*	*(4)*	*(5)*	*(6)*
Lactation tetany (grass staggers)	Hypomagnesaemia, hypocalcaemia, heavily fertilized pastures or with high potassium content	Ruminant	Tonic and clonic muscular spasms and convulsions. Death mostly due to respiratory failure.	Clinical findings and biochemistry with hypomagnesaemia and hypocalcaemia	Serum samples or uncoagulated blood.
Paralytic Myoglobin-uria (*Azoturia*)	Accumulation of lactic acid in muscles due to exercise after a period of idleness.	Horses	Signs occur 15 min. to 1 hour after exercise. Profuse sweating, stiffness and reluctance to move progressing to dog sitting position and lateral recumbency. Severe pain, polypnea, & deep red brown urine	Clinical findings, spectroscopy of urine to differentiate myoglobin from hemoglobin in urine. Polycythemia, elevated CPK and SGOT.	Urine and serum samples under refrigeration.
Parturient parasis (milk fever)	Hypocalcaemia, shortly after parturition	Cattle, sheep and swine	History of recent parturition, brief excitement, tetany, muscular tremor of head and limbs, anorexia shaking of head, protrusion of tongue with grinding of teeth. Depression, ataxia, lateral recumbency, hypothermia.	Clinical signs, Serum biochemistry revealing hypocalcaemia mainly with hypophosphatemia and hyper-magnecemia.	Serum samples /plasma or uncoagulated blood.

contd...

Table 5.6–Contd...

(1)	*(2)*	*(3)*	*(4)*	*(5)*	*(6)*
Post-parturient hemoglobin-uria.	Diets low in phosphorus, prolonged hypo-phosphatemia is a major predis-posing cause.	Dairy cows	Post parturient hemoglobinuria, weak-ness, inappetance, dehydration, jugular pulse augmented, pallor, icterus, tachycardia, fever, hemolytic anemia.	Demonstration of hemoglobinuria,, Heinz bodies in RBCs. Hematology with lowered Hb and total erythrocytic count.	Uncoagulated blood, blood smears and urine sample.
Pregnancy toxemia (fat cow syndrome)	Feed deprivation or increased energy demand resulting into mobilization of excessive fat from fat depots	Cattle and sheep	Disease occurs in fat cows within few days following parturition. Anorexia, sever ketosis, recumbency. Some exhibiting nervous signs like muscular tremor of head and neck, stary gaze, tachycardia and coma.	Clinical signs, demonstration of hypoglycemia initially and finally hyperglycemia, elevated SGOT and SDH, ketonuria and proteinuria.	Serum or blood sample and urine sample.

Table 5.7: Laboratory Diagnosis of Chemical Poisoning.

Disease (1)	*Causative Agent (2)*	*Species Affected (3)*	*Symptoms (4)*	*Diagnostic Tests (5)*	*Materials Required (6)*
Arsenic	Ingestion or percutaneous absorption of arsenic compounds commonly from dipping solutions, insecticidal or herbicidal sprays	Cattle, sheep and horse	Severe abdominal pain, salivation, restlessness, grinding of teeth, vomiting, ruminal atony, fetid diarrhea and clonic convulsions.	Detection of arsenic in urine, feces, milk, in hair and tissues.	Urine (1 litre), feces, milk or liver, kidney, skin, hair and alimentary tract wall.
Hydrocyanic Acid poisoning	Ingestion of plants with cynogenetic glucosides	Cattle	Quick death following dyspnea, restlessness, anxiety, clonic convulsions and bright red mucosa.	Detection of hydrocyanic acid in suspected material or ruminal contents with Sodium Picrate Paper test.	Ingesta, ruminal contents, blood and muscles.
Lead poisoning	Ingestion of lead compounds or feeds containing lead from environmental pollution	Cattle, sheep, goat, pig, horses	Staggers, muscle tremor of head and neck, champing of jaws frothing at mouth, salivation. Bellowing, rolling of eyes, tonic clonic convulsions, circling, abnormal gait, hyperesthesia, fetid diarrhea and death.	Detection of lead above normal in blood, urine, feces, milk and tissues. Estimation of ã aminolevulinic acid dehydratase	Blood, urine, feces, milk, liver, kidney, bones, alimentary tract contents and suspected material.

contd...

Table 5.7–Contd...

(1)	*(2)*	*(3)*	*(4)*	*(5)*	*(6)*
Mercury poisoning	Ingestion of organic mercurial compounds used as antifungal and or inhalation of mercuric vapour	Cattle, horse, sheep, pigs	Acute gastero-enteritis, vomiting (hememesis), severe diarrhea and nephrotoxicity with oligouria, increased heart and respiratory rate and convulsions.	Detection of mercury in feces, urine and source material.	Feces, urine, suspected material and kidneys.
Nitrate and Nitrite poisoning	Ingestion of nitrate or preformed nitrite from toxic forage, immature green oats, Rye hay, corn or sorghum fodder, turnip tops or water from deep wells.	Cattle, sheep and horses	Salivation, abdominal pain, vomiting, diarrhea, dyspnea, gasping, muscular tremor, staggering gait, severe cyanosis, rapid small weak pulse and terminal clonic convulsions.	Detection of nitrite in blood of live animals, met - hemoglobin levels. Nitrate or nitrite content of suspected materials and diphenylamine Blue Test.	Blood, suspected material.

Table 5.8: Laboratory Diagnosis of Some Important Poultry Diseases.

Disease (1)	*Causative Agent* (2)	*Species Affected* (3)	*Symptoms* (4)	*Diagnostic Tests* (5)	*Materials Required* (6)
Avian influenza	Orthomyxo virus	Poultry, ducks, turkeys, quails	Dullness, drowsiness, cynosis of comb and wattles, oedema of face, respiratory distress, nervous signs include blindness, convulsions and paralysis.	Replication and isolation in 9-11 days chick embryo in allantoic cavity. HA test after treatment with known RD antiserum.	Nasal and cloacal swabs on ice. Tracheal scrapings on ice. Formalin fixed portions of liver, spleen, brain, kidney, intestine and proventriculus.
Avian leucosis complex (ALC)	RNA virus from oncorna genus.	Adult poultry birds	Tumors of lymphoblastic cells, tumorus growth of lymphocytes of bursa, tumors in liver, spleen and may occur in lungs and ovary.	FAT. CFT, virus neutralization test, precipitation test, ELISA.	Serum samples, blood smears and smears from affected organs. Formalin fixed portions of organ with lesions.
Avian tuberculosis	Mycobacterium avium	Adult birds, (often backyard poultry).	Raised nodules in bone marrow and liver(60-90%) or in spleen(50-80%) or in lungs (30-50%). Nodules are yellowish white in colour and contain cheesy exudates.	Demonstration of acidfast bacteria in smears of nodules, Tuberculin test, Rapid agglutination test.	Fresh and fixed portions of spleen, bone marrow and serum samples.

contd...

Table 5.8–Contd...

(1)	*(2)*	*(3)*	*(4)*	*(5)*	*(6)*
Chronic respiratory disease(CRD)	Mycoplasma gallisepticum	4 -10 weeks old broilers	Sneezing, respiratory distress, eyes may show frothy exudates and conjectivitis.	Plate agglutination test, haemagglutination inhibition test, FAT and culture of the organism.	Trachea tied on both ends, pieces of trachea, lungs and air sacs in formalin.
Colisepticemia	E. coli	Chicks, broilers, ducks	Diarrhea, soiling of vent, depression, anorexia, lesions are pericarditis, peri-hepatitis, air saculitis.	Culture, isolation and identification of organism. Pathogenicity test by air sac inoculation in 3 week old chicks	Swabs from spleen, cloaca and heart blood on ice. Fresh and fixed portions of liver, spleen, air sacs and intestine.
Fowl cholera	Pasturella multocida	Ducks, geese, pigeons, pheasants and poultry	Loss of appetite, bluishness of combs, wattles, fever, discharge from nostrils, greenish diarrhea.	Demonstration of organism in blood smears. Subcuta-neous or intraperi-toneal inoculation of suspected material in mice or pigeon.	Blood smears, fresh blood and spleen on ice.
Infectious bronchitis	RNA corona virus	Poultry, common in baby chicks	Sneezing, respiratory rales, dyspnea, dull, huddling and diarrhea. Catarrhal or cheesy exudates in nasal cavity and adjoining sinuses. Both brochi display caseous plugs at entry point in lungs. Nephrosis may be there with deposition of urates.	Virus isolation in 9-12 day chick embryo in allantoic sac. FAT, ELISA, virus neutralization test	Trachea and lungs on ice, tracheal and lung swabs in transport medium, serum from convalescing birds.

Table 5.8–Contd...

(1)	(2)	(3)	(4)	(5)	(6)
Infectious bursal disease (IBD)	RNA virus	Chickens of 3-6 weeks.	Dullness, depression, trembling, ruffled feathers, watery diarrhea and prostration. Lesions include haemorrhages in skeletal muscles of leg and mucosa of proventriculus. Nephrosis, bursa swollen and edematous.	AGPT, ELISA, virus neutralization and isolation in chick embryo from spleen and bursal tissue inoculated in yolk sac or CAM.	Serum samples, bursa fabricius and kidney in transport medium. Portions of bursa and kidney in formal saline.
Infectious coryza	Haemophilus paragallinarum	Young adult birds	Exudation from nostrils and eyes, face and wattles swollen and dyspnea.	Demonstration of organism in smears of nasal or eye exudates, H.A test, culture, isolation & identification of organism.	Swabs from nose, trachea, orbital sinus on ice, smears of exudates, serum samples.
Infectious laryngo-tracheitis (ILT)	DNA herpes virus	Adult poultry birds.	Dyspnea, open mouth breathing, bluish wattles, sneezing, cough, rales, dull wet eyes and conjectivitis. Lesions include laryngeal and tracheal inflammation and congestion and some times with cheesy exudates.	Virus isolation, CAM inoculation of 10 day old chick embryos with tracheal scrapings results in formation of pocks after 3 days. AGPT, FAT, virus neutralization and histopathology.	Fresh pieces of trachea, air sacs and lungs in transport medium. Formalin fixed pieces of trachea, air sac and lungs. Serum samples and smears from mucosa of trachea.

contd...

Table 5.8–Contd...

(1)	*(2)*	*(3)*	*(4)*	*(5)*	*(6)*
Marek's disease (MD)	DNA herpes virus group B	Poultry, rarely turkeys and pheasants.	Dullness, respiratory distress, lameness or paralysis of one or both legs or wings, torticolitis. Lesions include thickening of sciatic nerves or brachial or vagus nerves.	AGPT, FAT, virus neutralization, and isolation in 5-6 day old chick embryo in yolk sac.	Affected nerves in formalin, serum samples from sick birds and feather follicles.
Newcastle disease (ND)	Paramyxo virus	Poultry and flying birds.	Loss of appitite, closed eyes, drooping wings, diarrhea, respiratory distress, twitching of neck and paralysis. Lesions include haemorrhagic ulcers in intestine, caecal tonsils and proventricular glands.	Virus isolation from bone marrow or spleen tissues, H.A & H.I test, FAT,CFT and virus neutralization.	Liver, spleen or brain in 50% glycerin saline. Fixed portions of proventriculus and brain.

contd...

Table 5.8–Contd...

(1)	(2)	(3)	(4)	(5)	(6)
Salmonellosis Paratyphoid	Salmonella typhimurium, S. enteridis.	2-4 week old chicks.	Loss of appetite, fever, white or yellowish diarrhea, huddling near the source of heat, drooping of wings. Lesions include enlargement of liver and spleen with necrotic spots and enteritis.	Isolation and identification of organism. Plate and tube agglutination test. Symptoms and age of affected birds.	Faecal samples, fresh and fixed portions of liver and spleen. Serum samples from ailing and recovered birds.
Pullorum	S. pullorum	Newly hatched chicks.			
Fowl typhoid	S. gallinarum	Adult birds of 3-6 months.			
Spirochetosis	Borrelia anserina	Poultry and turkeys	Greenish diarrhea, depression, loss of appetite, cyanosis of comb, anaemia. In coordinating movements and paralysis. Necropsy reveals very large spleen with molted appearance.	Demonstration of spirochaetes in blood smears or spleen impression smears. Culture of the organisms in yolk sac of 6 day old chick embryo. AGPT and FAT.	Blood smear, spleen impression smears, fresh and fixed portions of spleen and liver.

Table 5.9: Morphological, Biochemical and Cultural Characteristics of Pathogenic Organisms Commonly Associated with Animal Diseases.

Organism (1)	General Characteristics (2)	Cultural Characteristics (3)	1	2	3	4	5	6	7	8	9	10	11	12	13	14	15	16	17	18	19
Actinobacillus	Small, rod or Cocco-bacillary and aerobic	Blood agar, Nutrient agar (viscous, sticky colony) and Broth (turbidity & small deposit)	-	-	-			+	+	-	+	+	+		+		-	±		+	±
Actinomyces	Short, pleomorphic rods to branching filaments, anaerobic, growth enhanced with CO_2	Blood agar (raised, nodular colony, firmly adherent to medium)Brain Heart Infusion agar.	+		-	-	+	-	+	±	-		+	±	-						
Bacillus anthracis	Large selendrical rod, short chains, aerobic, central spore.	Nutrient agar (opaque medusa head colony) Blood agar(slight hemolysis)	+	+	-	+	+	-	+	-	-	+	+	+				+	-		
Brucella	Small, cocco-bacillary rod, aerobic, nonspore forming, Requires 5-10% CO_2 for growth.	Serum dextrose agar(delicate,semi-transparent colony), Tryptose agar, Liver infusion serum agar, potato agar. Colonies may be smooth, rough or mucoid.	-	+	-	-											-	-	-		±

contd...

Table 5.9–Contd...

(1)	(2)	(3)	1	2	3	4	5	6	7	8	9	10	11	12	13	14	15	16	17	18	19
Clostredium chauvoei	Rod, singly or short chain. Elongated, oval, sub-terminal or terminal spores, anaerobic	Simple media with glucose, Heart meat infusion or Liver extract. Blood agar (whitish gray colony, irregular zone of hemolysis)	+	-	+	+	+	+	+	-		+	+				-	-	-		
Cl. septicum	Rod, singly or short chain. Elongated, oval, sub-terminal or terminal spores, anaerobic	Simple media with glucose, Heart meat infusion or Liver extract. Blood agar (whitish gray colony, irregular zone of hemolysis)	+	-	+	+	+	+	-	+	-	+	+	+	-	+	-	-	-		+
Cl. tetani	Long slender rod, terminal spores, drum-stick like, anaerobic	Liquid media with meat particles or agar	+	-	+	+	-	-	-			-				-					
Cl. botulinum	Large bacillus in pairs or chains or singly, spores ova, terminal or sub-terminal.	Alkaline medium (large colony with irregular edges), Horse blood agar (hemolysis), Cooked meat media (blackened)	+	-	+	+	+	-	-			+							-		
Compylobactor (vibrio)	Comma or S shaped, spiral forms, requires 10% CO_2 for growth.	Blood agar (fine pin point bluish), Serum agar, Semisolid agar medium.	-		+									+	+				-		±

contd...

Table 5.9–Contd...

(1)	(2)	(3)	1	2	3	4	5	6	7	8	9	10	11	12	13	14	15	16	17	18	19
Corynebacterium	Small coccoid, pleomorphic, arranged in bundles or clusters, aerobic or facultative anaerobic. Metachromatic granules visible on staining.	Blood agar (hemolysis), Serum agar (dew drop coloy)	+	-	-	+	+	+	-	-	-	+		±	+	+	-	-	-		
Erysipelothrix	Short, selender rod, non-sporing, aerobic or facultative anaerobic	Blood agar (slight hemolysis) Nutrient agar(small, glistering, translucent colony)	+	-	-		+	+					+	-	-	+	-	-	-		+
Escherichia coli	Short rod, non-sporing, aerobic.	Mac.Conkey agar (large pink colony) Nutrient agar (low convex, smooth colourless colony) Broth (cloudiness) EMB(metallic sheen)	-	+	+	-	+	+	+		+						+	-	+		-
Haemophilus	Short coccoid, pleomorphic bacilli, occurring singly or in pairs or in short chains, non-spore forming	No growth on ordinary medium. Heated Blood agar (small, translucent, droplet like colony at 2-3 days incubation)	-	+	-		+								±				±	-	

contd...

Table 5.9–Contd...

(1)	*(2)*	*(3)*	*1*	*2*	*3*	*4*	*5*	*6*	*7*	*8*	*9*	*10*	*11*	*12*	*13*	*14*	*15*	*16*	*17*	*18*	*19*
Klebsiella	Thick rod, non motile, aerobic or facultative anaerobic	Solid agar (mucoid, moist, glistering, amorphous and opaque colony). In broth heavy turbidity.	-	+	-	-	+	+	+	+	+						-	+	±		-
Leptospira	Long, thin but closely spiraled with hooked ends, aerobic demonstrated in dark ground illumination with active movement in fresh preparations.	Protein rich semisolid or fluid medium, Rabbit serum enriched medium Fletcher's agar or Korthof"s medium. Incubation for six weeks. Intra perito-neal inoculation of hamsters or G.pigs.			+																
Listeria	Small rod with rounded ends, aerobic or micro-aerophilic may be in chains. Coccoid in tissue smears.	Tryptose agar (fine, blue green colony) Blood agar (small, rounded colony with β hemolysis)	+	-	+		+		+	+	-	+	+		+			+			-
Moraxella	Rod or cocco-bacillary, paired, aerobic and nonspore forming.	Blood agar (small, translucent, grayish white colony with zone of hemolysis) Chocolate agar. Peptone broth-(granular deposit)	-	+	-	±	-	-				-		+		+				+	

contd...

Table 5.9–Contd...

(1)	(2)	(3)	1	2	3	4	5	6	7	8	9	10	11	12	13	14	15	16	17	18	19
Mycobacterium	Slim rod, aerobic, nonsporing, acid fast, is occurring singly or in pairs or bundles.	Dorset egg medium with 4-5 days incubation. Jensen medium with 3-6 weeks incubation, raised, adherent colony & buff pigment. Liquid medium enriched with bovine serum, albumin and casein hydrolysate.	ACID FAST	-										±							
Mycoplasma	Organism do not possess cell wall, have triple layered membrane having sterols, contains DNA & RNA, no nuclear membrane. Aerobic, some require 10% Co_2. During life cycle variety of granules or cocci develop referred as elementary bodies, clubs, filaments, rings or satellite forms. Diene's staining for colonies on agar.	Growth in heart infusion peptone containing 20% horse serum, 10% yeast extract, 20ug DNA, 50iu pencillin,0.25 mg thalous acetate per ml. Incubation at 37°C for 48-96 hrs. On mycoplasma agar colonies are round, granular surface, dark centre buried in agar, visible only by low power microscope. Inoculation in 7 day's chick embryo via yolk sac. Tissue cultures are also in use now-a-days.																			

contd...

Table 5.9–Contd...

(1)	(2)	(3)	1	2	3	4	5	6	7	8	9	10	11	12	13	14	15	16	17	18	19
Pasteurella multocida	Coccobacillary, pleomorphic, bipolar, aerobic or facultative anaerobic, nonspore forming.	Nutrient agar (small round flat mucoid colony). Blood or serum enriched medium. No growth on Mac- Conkey's medium.	-	+	-	-	+	-	+		+	-		+					+	+	+
Pasteurella hemolytica	Coccobacillary, pleomorphic, bipolar, aerobic or facultative anaerobic, nonspore forming.	Blood or serum agar (small, round, moist colony) weekly hemolytic. Growth on MacConkey's medium.	-	+	-	-	+	+		-	+	+		+					-	+	+
Pseudomonas aeruginosa	Slender rod, aerobic, nonspore forming. Produces bluish green pig-ment (pyocyanin) in medium.	Nutrient agar (large, irregular, translucent colony with entire or undulate edges).In broth thick pellicle is formed.	-	-	+	+	+	-				-		-			-	-		+	-
Pseudomonas mallei	Slender rod with rounded ends, may be coccoid, non spore forming, aerobic or faculata-tive anaerobic.	Glycerin agar (small, amorphous, round, translucent, slimy colony). Colonies become yellowish brown when it ages.	-	-	-		+					-		-			-	-	-	-	+

contd...

Table 5.9–Contd...

(1)	(2)	(3)	1	2	3	4	5	6	7	8	9	10	11	12	13	14	15	16	17	18	19
Pneumococcus	Diplococci, aerobic or facultative anaerobic, growth in 5-10% Co_2	Blood agar (flat, moist,transparent colony, α hemolysis)	+	±	-			+	+		-			+							
Proteus	Bacilli displaying pleomorphism, nonspore forming and fimbriate, aerobic or facultative anaerobic. Seminal odour and swarming are characteristics.	Growth in ordinary medium with discrete colonies only in early stages of incubation and thereafter a thin film of growth on medium due to swarming .	-	-	+	+	+	-	±	-	-						+	-	+		+
Salmonella	Rod shaped, fimbriate, aerobic or facultative anaerobic, nonspore forming	Nutrient agar (round, (smooth colony) MacConkey's agar (pale, white colony) Deoxy-cholate agar (black colony). S.S agar, EMB agar, selenite or tetrathionate broths are selective media.	-	+	+	-	+	-	-	-	+						+	-	-		+
Shigella	Rod shaped, aerobic or facultative anaerobic, nonspore forming	MacConkey's agar and DCA agar (pink colony)	-		-	-	-	-	-	-	±						+	-	±		-

contd...

Table 5.9–Contd...

(1)	(2)	(3)	1	2	3	4	5	6	7	8	9	10	11	12	13	14	15	16	17	18	19
Staphylococcus	Spherical cocci , forming grape like clusters, aerobic, non-sporing. Produce pigments with colour varying from white to yellow.	Nutrient agar (soft, entire, low, convex, pigmented colony) Blood agar (β hemolysis) MacConkey's agar (small pink yellow or deep red colony)	+		-	+	+	+	+	-	+	+		+	+	+	+	+	-	-	
Streptococcus	Oval, spherical forming chains, aerobic or facultative anaerobic, non-spore forming.	Blood agar (circular, grayish, mucoid colony with α or β hemolysis). Poor growth on MacConkey's agar.	+	±	±		+	+		+	±				-					-	
Yersina pseudo-Tuberculosis	Coccobacillary, pleo-morphic,aerobic or facultative anaerobic.	MacConkey's agar (round, umbonate, buttery colony).In broth forms pellicle.	-		+		+	-		+	+	+	+	+					-		
Rickettsia	Short pleomorphic. Cell membrane and cell wall present. Do not grow in artificial medium. Growth in living cells. Obligate inter-cellular parasites.	Yolk sac inoculation in chick embryos and intraperitoneal inoculation of guinea pigs, rabbits, mice or hamsters.	-																		

1. Gram's staining, 2. Capsule, 3. Motility, 4. Gelatin liquefaction, 5. Gluccse, 6. Lactose, 7. Sucrose, 8. Salicin, 9. Manitol, 10. Maltose, 11. Fructose, 12. Nitrate reduction, 13. catalase, 14. Coagulase, 15. Methyl red, 16. Voges-Proskauer, 17. Indole, 18. Oxidase, 19. Hydrogen sulphide. (+ = positive, - = negative, ± = some strains positive and some negative)

Table 5.10: Morphological and Cultural Characteristics of Viruses Associated with Animal Diseases.

Virus	*Morphological Characteristics*	*Cultural Characteristics*
Adenovirus	Non-enveloped, double stranded DNA, multiplies in nucleus with formation of basophilic or acidophilic inclusion bodies.	Cultured in cell cultures of calf kidney or testicle cells from natural or closely related species. CPE is characterized by rounding and clumping of affected cells as bunching of grapes. Avian adenoviruses are propagated in chicken embryos causing death and stunting growth of embryos. Chicken embryo kidney, liver or fibroblast cells support growth and produce CPE with intra nuclear inclusions.
Bunyavirus	Medium sized, enveloped. single stranded RNA virus, replicates in cytoplasm. Some viruses induce cell fusion and intra nuclear inclusions.	Growth in cell cultures and lab mice. Isolation in the brain of suckling mouse of 1-2 days age. Can be cultivated in primary cell cultures as well as in continuous cell cultures with production of CPE.
Calcivirus	Spherical, non-enveloped RNA virus, replicates in cytoplasm.	Growth in embryonic kidney cells from the species of origin.
Herpes virus BHV-1 & BHV – 2	Large180-200nm, enveloped, linear double stranded DNA virus, replicates in nucleus and leaves it by budding from the nuclear membrane.	Multiplies in a wide variety of cell cultures, however, isolation is better in bovine kidney or testes cell cultures with CPE characterized by rounding of cells, refractile and formation of syncytia and intranuclear inclusions. Do not grow in embryonated eggs.

contd...

Table 5.10–Contd...

Virus	*Morphological Characteristics*	*Cultural Characteristics*
Marek's disease virus	DNA virus with two types, one naked and second enveloped. Enveloped virion of MDV have two types, one found in nucleus of infected cells, presumed to be non infectious and other in the cytoplasm, is infectious. All the isolated strains of virus have been found antigenically homogenous.	Virus cultivated in susceptible chicks, chick embryos and cell cultures. Inoculation of day old chicks with suspected material results into development of lesions in ganglia, nerves with mononuclear infiltration around nerves after 2-3 weeks. Propagation of virus in chick embryo via CAM or yolk sac rote with formation of discrete white pocks on CAM. Virus can be grown in cell cultures of chicken kidney and duck embryo fibroblast with production of CPE characterized by rounded and fusiform refractile cells and polykaryocytes with inclusions in nucleus.
Newcastle disease virus	Relatively large, enveloped with haemagglutinin, neuraminidase and fusion protein. It is potant inducer of interferon.	Cultured in chick embryo with allantoic cavity inoculation. Most of the strains kill embryo within 24 to 72 hours causing haemorrhagic lesions and encephalitis. Also replicates in cell culture systems like chick embryo fibroblast, chick, rabbit, pig, calf or monkey kidney and BHK-21 and Hela cells with production of poly-karyocytes in infected cells.
Orthomyxo-virus (influenza viruses)	Type A influenza virus is roughly spherical or filamentous, enveloped, single stranded RNA virus having both haemagglutinin and neuraminidase.	Growth in 10 days old chick embryo in amniotic or allantoic cavity. Some isolates replicate in cell cultures producing CPE as rounding and detachment of cells.

contd...

Table 5.10–Contd...

Virus	*Morphological Characteristics*	*Cultural Characteristics*
Papillomavirus	Non-enveloped, icosahedral,double stranded DNA, relatively resistant virus.	Subcutaneous inoculation in un-weaned hamsters or mice results in the development of tumors at the inoculation site within 100 days. Virus can produce non-productive infections in embryonic cells of hamsters, mice and cattle with cellular transformation. Does not grow in chick embryo.
Parvovirus	Non-enveloped, single stranded DNA molecule. Some strains haemagglutinate RBCs and some produce CPE.	Virus grows in young actively growing pig primary kidney cell cultures, testicular, thyroid, foetal kidney and continuous cell lines with production of CPE and intra-nuclear inclusions.
Paramyxovirus	Spherical, enveloped, single stranded, un-segmented RNA virus. It has three genera as (1) Paramyxovirus having haemagglutinin and neuraminidase, (2) Morbillivirus containing haemagglutinin but no neuraminidase, (3) Pneumovirus having neither haemagglutinin nor neuraminidase.	Growth in chick embryo and tissue cultures. CPE characterized by formation of inclusion bodies and syncytial formation followed by death and detachment. Marbillivirus replicates in primary and continuous dog and ferret kidney cells or in chick embryo fibroblast with CPE including granular degeneration and vacuolation of cells and formation of giant cells and syncytia including cytoplasmic and nuclear inclusions.
Pestivirus (BVD virus)	Spherical, enveloped, single stranded RNA virus. Few agglutinate monkey, guinea pig, sheep or chicken RBCs.	Growth in tissue cultures derived from chick embryo, mouse, hamster, monkey or guinea pigs with production of CPE. Several strains do not produce CPE. Certain strains grow in yolk sac of chick embryo. Propagation also in embryonated eggs causing haemorrhage and death of embryo in 24-48 hours.

contd...

Table 5.10–Contd...

Virus	*Morphological Characteristics*	*Cultural Characteristics*
Picorna virus	Small, nacked, single stranded RNA virus. It includes entero, rhino, cardio and aphtho viruses. FMD virus has antigenic variation with serotypes O,A,C, ASIA-1, SAT-1, SAT-2, and SAT-3	Growth in cell cultures producing CPE characterized by granularity and rounding of affected cells with complete destruction in 48-72 hours. FMD virus propagates by intradermal inoculation of guinea pig foot pads and lesions develop within 24-48 hours at the site of inoculation. Replication in a number of trypsinized cell culture systems like bovine tongue epithelium, bovine thyroid, bovine embryo, rabbit embryo lungs, calf, pig, lamb and goat kidney with production of CPE.
Pox viruses	Large brick shaped or ovoid, 300-450nm x 170-260nm ,enveloped containing single molecule of double stranded DNA. There are about ten major antigens and one antigen cross reacts with the most pox viruses of vertebrates. Multiplies in the cytoplasm and produce 'B' & 'A type inclusions.	Most of pox viruses grow in embryonated eggs and produce pocks on the chorioallantoic membrane, can also be cultivated in cell cultures like chicken embryo fibroblasts, bovine or rabbit kidney or Hela cells. CPE is produced with formation of giant cells, basophilic and oesinophilic inclusions in the cytoplasm.
Reo virus	Virus usually naked, may have pseudomembranes of host origin, double stranded RNA, comprising of 10-12 segments. agglutinate human "O" RBCs. Replication in cytoplasm with production of inclusions.	Bovine strains are isolated in monkey kidney cells with production of eosinophilic inclusions in the cytoplasm of infected cells. Avian reoviruses grow readily in chick embryo by yolk sac or chorio-allantoic membrane inoculation resulting into death of embryo between 3-8 days and formation of small white pocks on CAM. Virus also replicates in cell cultures of vero cells or chick embryos.

contd...

Table 5.10–Contd...

Virus	*Morphological Characteristics*	*Cultural Characteristics*
Rhabdo virus	Oblong with one round and one planer end looks like a bullet, enveloped, linear single stranded RNA virus. Cytoplasmic replication with formation of inclusion bodies.	Intracerebral inoculation in mammals particularly dog or rabbit is adopted to get laboratory or fixed virus where as virus isolated from clinical cases is called street virus. Suckling mouse or 5-6 days embryonated eggs are now commonly used. Virus isolation in tissue cultures has been tried with poor CPE.
Rinderpest virus	Spherical or ovoid, some are filamentous and elongated, enveloped virus with large projections, relatively fragile.	Grows well in primary or continuous cell cultures from cattle, sheep, goat, chick embryo, pig, hamsters, dog and man with production of CPE characterized by multinucleated giant cells or syncytia and intranuclear inclusions.
Rota virus	Virus particle measures about 70-75nm, consists of central core surrounded by two layers of virus specific polypeptides. Double stranded RNA segments.	Difficult to propagate in cell cultures, have been adopted to grow in bovine and simian kidney cultures. Isolation and cultivation is facilitated by treatment of faecal samples with trypsin and pancreatin.
Toga virus	Spherical, enveloped, single stranded RNA virus. Agglutinates chicken RBCs.	Growth in tissue cultures derived from chick embryo, mouse, hamster, monkey or guinea pigs with production of CPE. Propagation also in embryonated eggs causing haemorrhage and death of embryo in 24-48 hours.
Visna/maedi virus	Spherical, enveloped, linear single stranded RNA virus. Does not show haemagglutination properly but inhibits haemagglutination by influenza virus.	Virus propagation in sheep cell cultures with production of syncytia and cellular degeneration. Growth in BHK-21 cells and primary cell cultures of bovine, porcine, canine or human choride plexus cells. No growth in chick embryos.

Chapter 6

Special Laboratory Techniques

Agar Gel Precipitation Test

The gels of agar or gelatin are used for demonstration of precipitation reactions for assay purposes. The test is based on the principle that when an antigen solution is layered on top of serum containing specific antibodies or precipitins against the antigen, a ring of white precipitate is formed.

A very simple and common technique of allowing antigen and antibody to diffuse towards each other is demonstrated best in a plate of agar gel in which the wells are cut. In this technique not only one test antigen but several test antigens may be placed in wells around a central well of known antiserum and the number of precipitation lines formed by antigen antibody diffusion will indicate the number of antigens in each solution. Gel diffusion precipitation can be used not only for quantitative and qualitative assays of antigens or antibodies, in many bacterial and viral diseases, but also to detect the presence of diffusible toxins in cultures.

1. 1% agar is dissolved in 0.01 M phosphate buffer saline with or with out glycerin 7.5%.
2. The mixture is autoclaved at 15 lbs pressure for 20 minutes.
3. Melted agar is poured on glass slides or Petri dish.
4. Wells are punched or dug in the agar at a distance of 3 to 4mm.
5. Antigen is filled in one well and antiserum in other well with the help of a pasture pipette.
6. Charged slides are kept at 37^{0}C in a Petri dish with wet filter papers to avoid desiccation.

7. Slides are examined for precipitation bands against a beam of light at every 12 hours for 3 to 5 days.

Ascoli Precipitin Test

Anthrax, a very acute disease of livestock, has a short incubation period and duration with no specific antibody response of the host that can be used an index of infection. However in recovered animals demonstration of toxin neutralizing antibodies in the serum may be of value.

Ascoli devised a test for the detection of soluble anthrax antigens, extractable from infected tissues with saline. The test is of a certain value as an ancillary means of diagnosis, especially where animal is in advanced decomposition and culture of organism would be impossible. This method involves mixing of immunized rabbit serum with an extract of test organs for observation of precipitate formation.

Procedure

1. Grind the organs or blood of suspected animal.
2. Suspend it in saline.
3. Boil it for 5 minutes.
4. Filter through filter paper and allow it to cool.
5. Stratify carefully 0.5ml of this filtrate on 0.5ml immune serum in small test tubes.
6. Allow the tubes to stand at room temperature for15 minutes.
7. A ring like precipitate is formed at the junction of two in positive cases.
8. Always keep controls with known anthrax.

Chick Embryo Inoculation Techniques

The fairly common method of virus inoculation is chick embryo inoculation. It requires;

1. Live embryonated eggs exhibiting a well defined blood vessel pattern and active motility.
2. An egg incubator or simple incubator can be used with placement of water tray in it to maintain humidity and prevent desiccation of eggs.

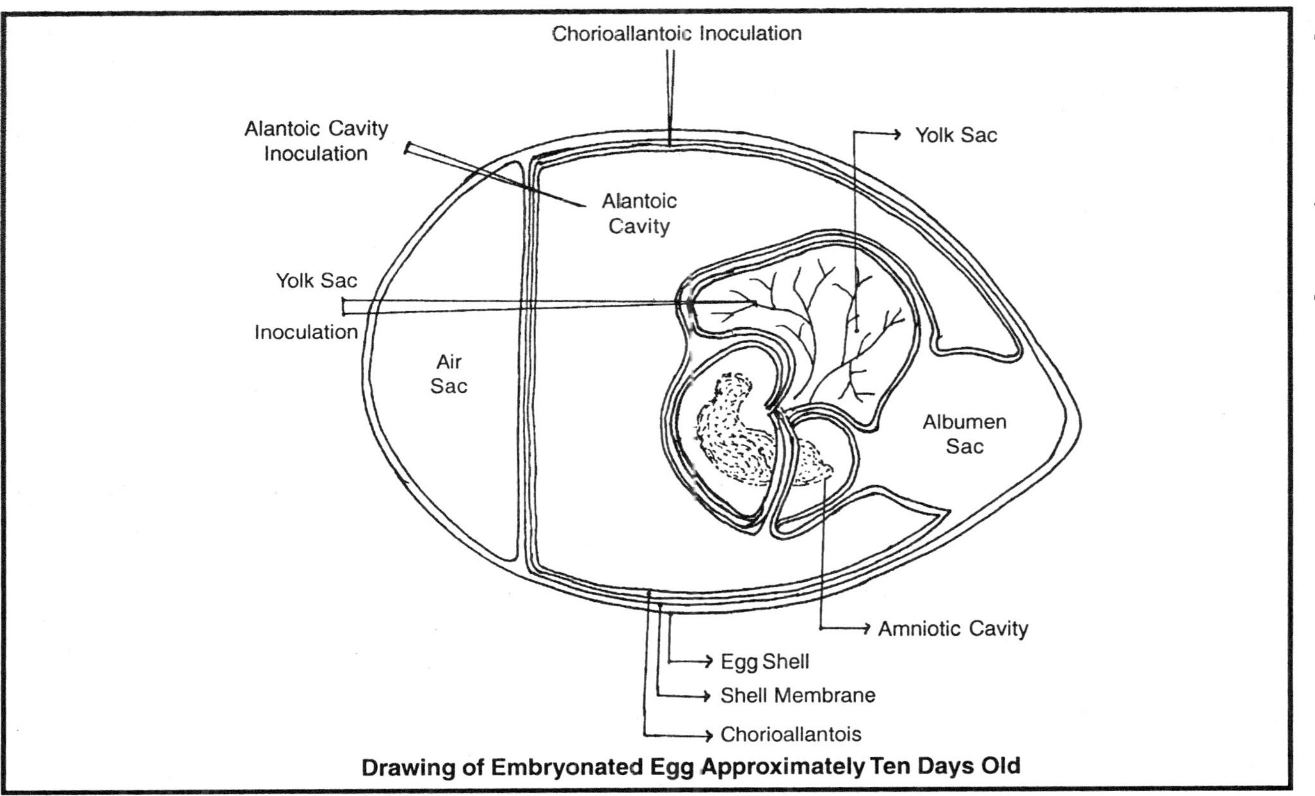

Drawing of Embryonated Egg Approximately Ten Days Old

3. A candler
4. A hand drill
5. Egg trays
6. Inoculating syringes (sterile)

The age of embryos to be used for inoculation largely depend upon the route of inoculation.

Chorio-allantoic Membrane Inoculation

1. Wipe the egg surface with betadine or 70% alcohol.
2. Treat the material to be inoculated with streptomycin and penicillin(500mg and 500 iu per ml respectively).
3. Candle 10 – 12 days old embryonated eggs for viability of embryo.
4. Select live embryos and chalk out the air sac with a marker pen.
5. Cut a triangular flap or a groove with the help of an electric drill or small glass saw over the centre of air sac.
6. Cut a second flap or groove over the centre of egg through the shell avoiding chorio-allantoic membrane.
7. Put the egg over candler in horizontal position and apply suction at the air sac end of the egg with the help of a rubber bulb.
8. Observe the movement of embryo into the air sac and disappearance of blood vessels adjacent to shell membrane and formation of a new air sac under lateral slit or groove.
9. Inoculate the material onto chorio-allantoic membrane by piercing lateral slit and allowing needle to go just under the shell membrane.
10. Cover the slits with melted paraffin wax or cello tape.
11. Incubate the eggs at 37°C for required time, generally 48-72 hours.
12. Candle the eggs at 24 hours of inoculation for viability and discard any deaths within 24 hours of inoculation.
13. Cut the shell over the false air sac starting from lateral slit.
14. Grasp the chorio-allantoic membrane with pair of forceps near edge of the shell.

15. Cut an oval area of the chorio-allantoic membrane and place it in a Petri dish containing saline solution.
16. Place the Petri dish on a black surface and observe the membrane for viral growth.
17. Edema and thickening of membrane with large areas of opacity, discrete pock like lesions varying in size from 1mm plaques to large plaques, represents the viral growth.

Allantoic Cavity Inoculation

1. Wipe the egg surface with betadine or 70% alcohol.
2. Treat the material to be inoculated with streptomycin and penicillin (500mg and 500 iu per ml respectively).
3. Candle 10 – 12 days old embryonated eggs for viability of embryo.
4. Select live embryos and chalk out the air sac with a marker pen.
5. Drill a hole just above the air sac through shell membrane in to air sac.
6. Inoculate by inserting a 24 gauge, 3/4inch long needle vertically through the hole directly in to the allantoic cavity.
7. Seal the inoculation site with paraffin wax or cello tape or nail polish.
8. Incubate the eggs at 37°C for 40-48 hours.
9. Candle the eggs for viability and discard the dead embryos.
10. Put eggs in the refrigerator for several hours to chill and kill the embryos so as to prevent bleeding at harvesting the fluid.
11. Place the chilled egg in holder with air sac end upwards and swab the shell with betadine or 70% alcohol.
12. Cut the shell over air sac and expose the allantoic fluid by tearing shell membrane and allantoic membrane with the help of sterile pointed forceps.
13. Suck out the fluid carefully by using pipette attached to suction pump or a rubber bulb
14. About 3-8ml of fluid can be collected, which is clear, though a heavy precipitate of amorphous urates may be present.
15. Presence of virus in the fluid can be detected by appropriate

tests like HA test, Macchiavello's staining or laboratory animal inoculation.

Yolk Sac Inoculation

1. Clean the egg surface with betadine or 70% alcohol.
2. Treat the material to be inoculated with streptomycin and penicillin (500mg and 500 iu per ml respectively).
3. Candle 5 - 8 days old embryonated eggs for viability of embryos.
4. Select live embryos and mark the area of embryo with a marker pen.
5. Drill a hole over the centre of air sac.
6. With 21 gauge, 1.5 inch long needle inject the material into the egg away from embryo.
7. Seal the slit with paraffin wax or cello tape or nail polish
8. Incubate the eggs at 37°C.
9. Candle the eggs for viability twice a day starting from second day after inoculation.
10. Harvest the yolk sac when eggs are enfeebled, indicated by sluggish movements of embryo.
11. Cut the shell over air sac and remove the shell membrane and chorio-allantoic membrane
12. Empty the contents of egg into a Petri dish.
13. Remove the yolk sac with the help of forceps and take a piece of yolk sac while whipping off the yolk.
14. Macerate the tissue on a slide.
15. Stain the slide with Macchiavello's stain.
16. Virus particles appear as minute red cocci.

Amniotic Sac Inoculation

1. Clean the egg surface with betadine or 70% alcohol.
2. Treat the material to be inoculated with streptomycin and penicillin (500mg and 500 iu per ml respectively).
3. Candle 6 - 8 days (for mumps virus), 13 days(for influenza virus) old embryonated eggs for viability of embryos.

4. Select live embryos and locate the position of the embryonic eye.
5. Drill a slit above the eye, over the air space.
6. Place the egg over candler in a horizontal position.
7. Inoculate by inserting 25gauge, 1.5 inch long needle through the slit with a swift thrust towards the embryo.
8. Volume of inoculum should be approximately 0.1ml.
9. Seal the opening with paraffin wax or nail polish.
10. Incubate the eggs at 37°C in an incubator for 6-7 days for mumps virus isolation and 3-4 days for influenza virus isolation.
11. After incubation, chill the embryos before harvesting.
12. Cut the shell over the embryo while placing the egg in horizontal position.
13. Tear off the allantoic membrane and remove the allantoic fluid.
14. Grasp the exposed amniotic membrane with a pair of forceps and remove the fluid with the help of a capillary pipette.
15. Presence of virus can be determined by HA test.

Complement Fixation Test (CFT)

Complement is a thermo-labile constituent of serum and acts as a catalyst for a variety of antigen-antibody reactions. Antibody apparently combines firmly with bacterial antigen and complement then unites with antigen antibody complex. The antibody and complement have no independent combining affinity. It is believed that antibody acts by sensitizing the antigen to the action of complement and the complement is essential lytic agent. Complement causes red cell hemolysis when a red cell suspension is mixed with the corresponding antibody. It can be easily understood from the given reaction.

Antigen + Antibody → Agglutination and no lysis.

Antigen + Antibody + complement → lysis of antigen.

Antigen + complement → No lysis.

Complement fixation test is one of the most commonly used serological test employed with soluble or particulate antigens for the detection of either antigen or antibody. This test requires following inputs.

Haemolytic System

It is an indicator of presence of complement. It consists of red blood cells of a particular animal species, sheep or ox, sensitized with the corresponding haemolytic antibody raised in rabbits by 5 to 6 intravenous injections of 10% sheep or ox red cells at 5 days interval. The raised serum is heat inactivated to render it non-haemolytic itself and can bring lysis only in presence of a suitable complement. Haemolytic system = {1.5% sheep cell suspension} + {4 times the highest dilution of haemolysin showing complete haemolysis}. Thus fixation of complement is denoted by absence of lysis in the haemolytic system.

Complement

Fresh or specially preserved guinea pig serum (pooled serum from many guinea pigs) is used. It contains an active haemolytic complement for the red blood cells of sheep or ox sensitized with homologous haemolytic antibody. It is advisable to keep serum on ice throughout the experiment because the complement is unstable and deteriorates on keeping at ordinary temperature. Complement serum can be preserved at -30°C for few weeks or can be lyophilized.

Antigen

Antigens of many bacterial, viral and rickettsial diseases are commercially available.

Antigen Complement Mixture

It is prepared by taking 0.9ml of 1:30 dilution of complement to which is added drop by drop 0.1ml of 1:10 diluted antigen. Then dilute 1:10 antigen further to 1:1000 in 1:30 complement to form antigen complement mixture.

Procedure

1. Heat inactivate the test serum at 56°C for 30 minutes.
2. Take 0.1ml of serum in two tubes.
3. Add 0.5ml of antigen complement mixture to one tube and 0.5ml of 1:30 complement to other tube (serum control)
4. Mix the contents by shaking and place in ice box at 6-8°C for 15 to 18 hours.
5. Place the tubes in water bath at 37°C for 10 minutes.

6. Add 0.5ml of 0.75% sensitized sheep cell suspension (sensitized 15 minutes before using).
7. Mix by shaking and place in water bath at 37°C for 30 minutes.

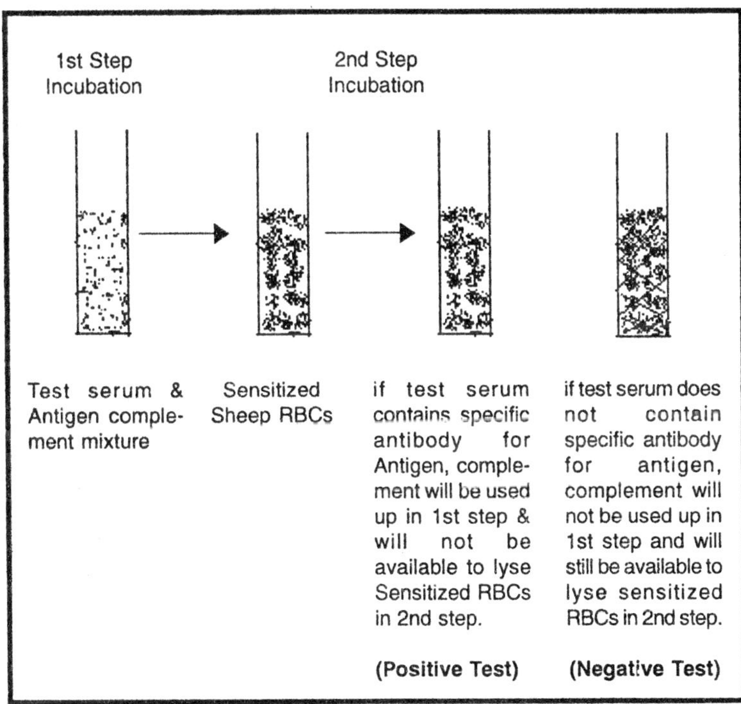

Camp Test

This test involves the completion of partial haemolysis (beta toxin zone) of *Staphylococcus aureus*, when *Streptococcus agalactiae* is streaked at right angles to Staphylococcus streaks on blood agar. The test may be conducted in a medium that contains beta toxins of *S.aureus* to screen for Streptococcus agalactiae. However, incorporation of esculin into the medium makes it possible to identify S.agalactiea, S. dysgalactiea and S. uberis by their ability or inability to hydrolyse esculin.

Use of Edward's medium containing esculin, crystal violet and thalium acetate may be of significant value in presumptive identification of important mastitis Streptococci. It inhibits Gram negative bacteria and staphylococcus.

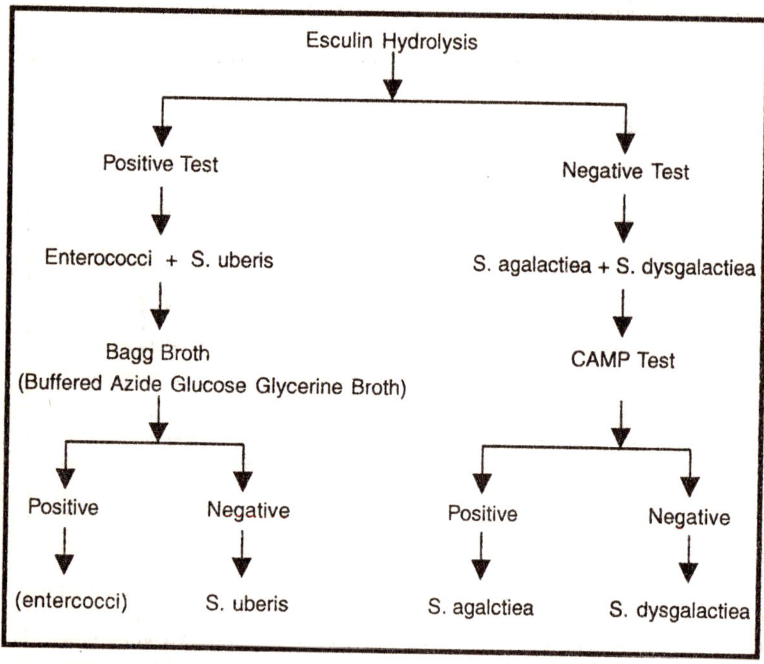

Enzyme Linked Immunosorbent Assay (ELISA)

The fact that proteins and lipopolysaccharides can passively be adsorbed to plastic has been exploited in the development of immunoassays and the immunoassay, involving the use of enzyme attached to one of the reagents utilized in the test, is termed as enzyme linked imunosorbent assay (ELISA). The resulting conjugates have both immunological and enzymatic activity. ELISA involves labeling of antigen or antibody with an enzyme and its binding to immunosorbent agent in ELISA plate that makes the antigen-antibody complex immobile and addition of relevant substrate chromogen solution causes a colour change that can be read both visually or by a spectrophotometer.

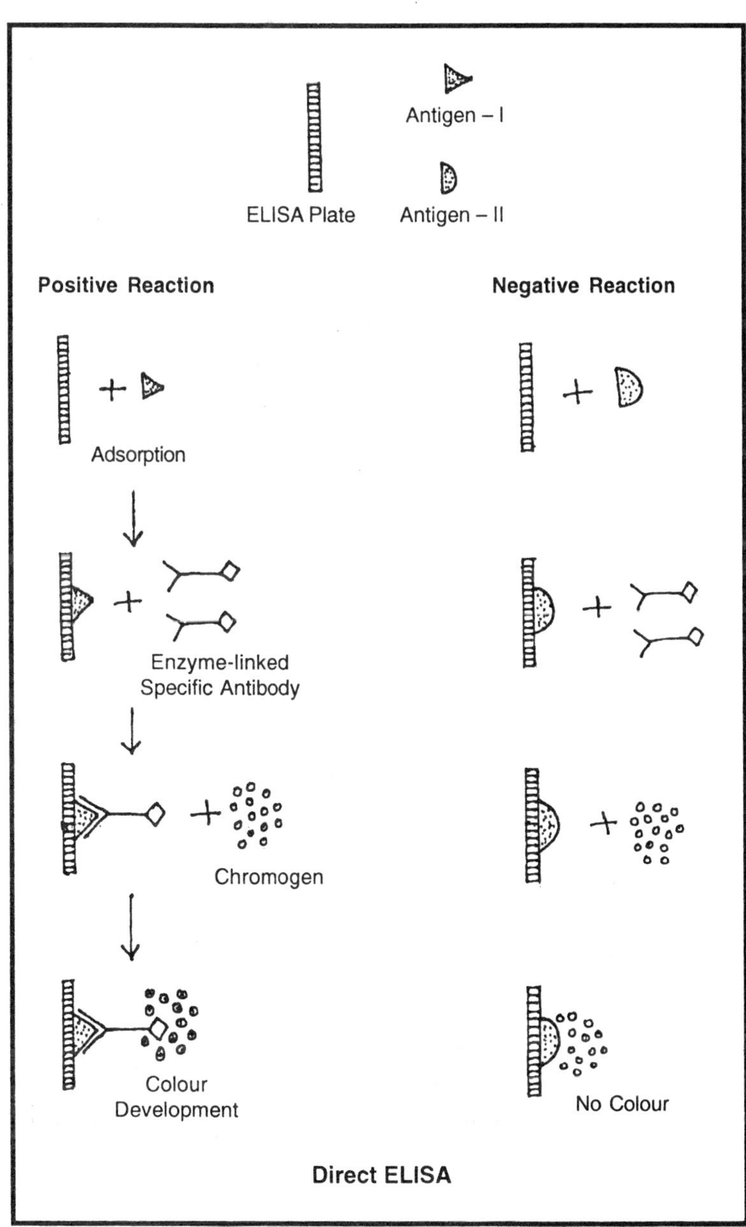

Direct ELISA

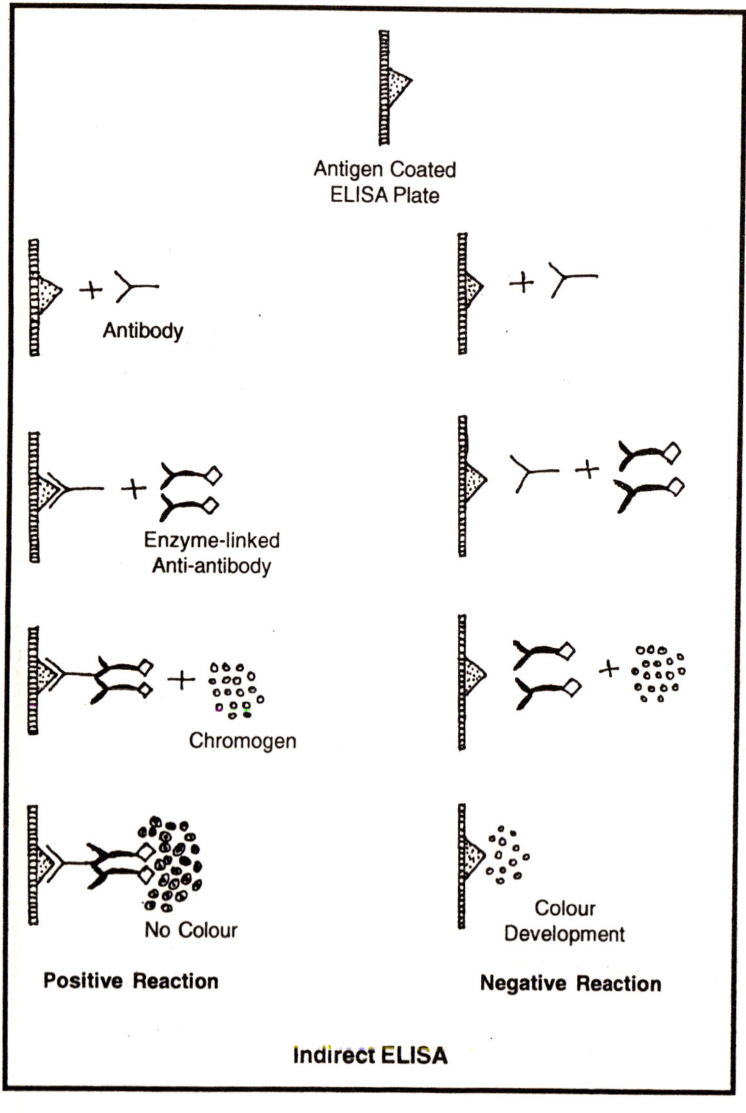

Indirect ELISA

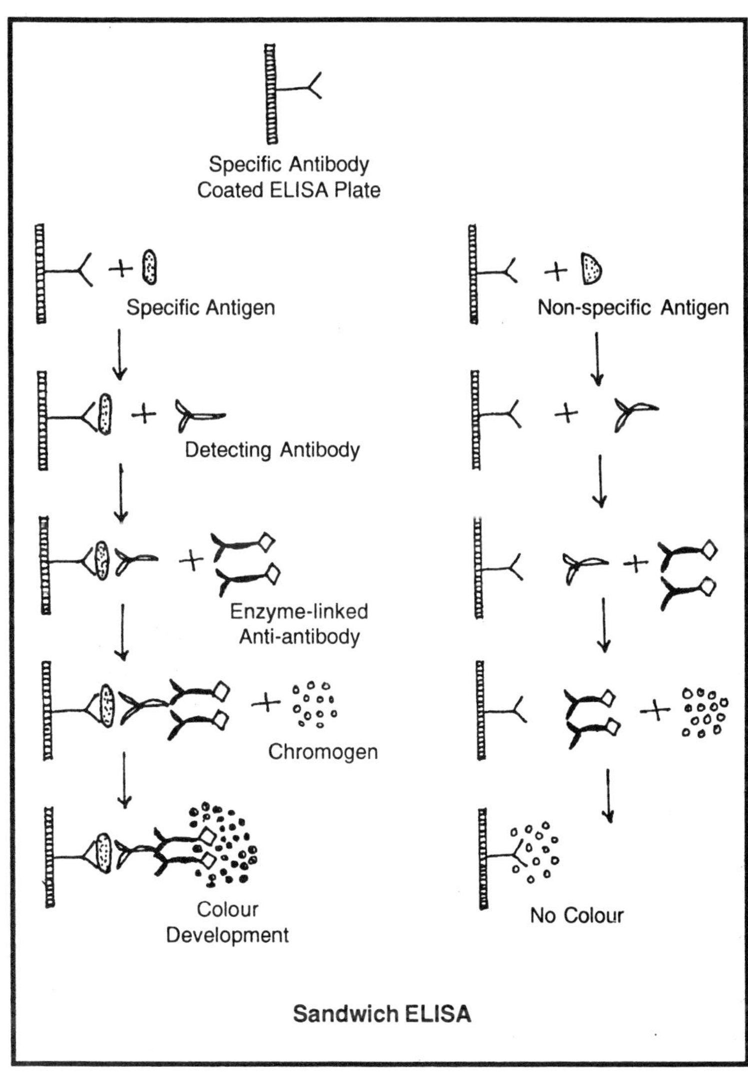
Specific Antibody
Coated ELISA Plate
Specific Antigen
Non-specific Antigen
Detecting Antibody
Enzyme-linked
Anti-antibody
Chromogen
Colour
Development
No Colour
Sandwich ELISA

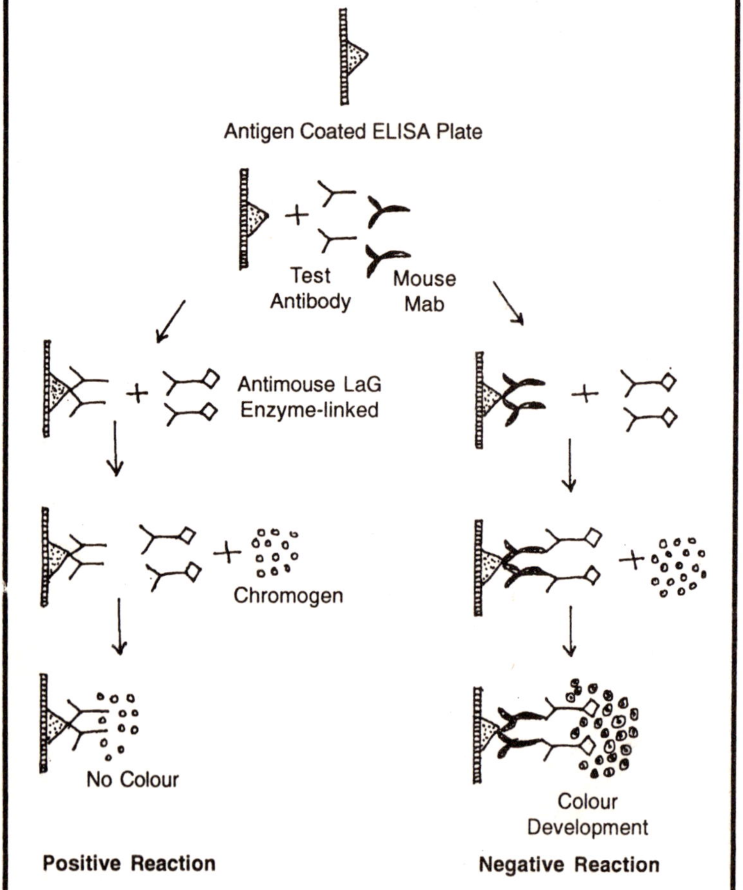

Antigen Coated ELISA Plate

Test Antibody

Mouse Mab

Antimouse LaG Enzyme-linked

Chromogen

No Colour

Colour Development

Positive Reaction

Negative Reaction

Competitive ELISA

ELISA test can be performed in different ways such as *Direct ELISA, Indirect ELISA, Sandwich ELISA or Competitive ELISA* that are best demonstrated in given flow charts.

ELISA Technique Requires Following Laboratory Facilities

1. ELISA Microplates, polyvinyl or polystyrene, 96 well with flat bottom,
2. Orbital shaker or microplate shaker.
3. Microplate washer automatic or simple plastic washbottle with suitable tubing.
4. Micropipettes single channel and multi-channel ranging from 5-50µl, 50-200µl, 200-1000µl.
5. Microplate ELISA reader with filters 492/405/450 nm.
6. Computer.
7. Freezer.
8. Incubator with microplate shaker fitted inside the incubator.

ELISA Test Involves Following Steps

Coating or Adsorption

1. Antigen + coating buffer is dispensed in wells of ELISA plate.
2. Incubation of plate at 37°C for 1 hour or at 4°C overnight.
3. Washing of plate with wash buffer atleast thrice.

Addition of Test and Control Sera

1. Add control and test sera to the designated coated wells.
2. Incubation is carried out for 1 hour at 37°C using plate shaker within the incubator.
3. Washing of plate with wash buffer thrice.

Addition of Conjugate

1. Enzyme labeled antibody or antigen as the case may be is added to each well.
2. Incubation is carried out for 1 hour.
3. Washing is made thrice with wash buffer.

Addition of Substrate and Chromogen

1. Appropriate substrate (hydrogen peroxide if peroxidase enzyme is labeled) along with chromogen is added to each well.
2. A clean uncoated plate is also charged with substrate and chromogen that serves as a blank.
3. Incubation is carried out for 15 minutes.

Stopping of Reaction

1. After suitable colour is developed add stopping solution like sulphuric acid.
2. Add the stopping solution to blank plate also.

Measuring of Optical Density

1. When the reaction is stopped, OD of blank is taken first from the ELISA reader and then the OD values of test plate is recorded.
2. Computer facility shall help in recording and interpreting the results.

Egg Counting in Faecal Sample

The only technique of faecal examination for both qualitative and quantitative diagnosis is direct saline smear or cellophane covered thick smear.

Direct Smear Egg Counts

The eggs are counted in a direct smear or in known quantity of faeces which can be facilitated by use of photoelectric light meter. The turbidity of test smear for knowing the quantity of faeces used can be compared with the turbidity of standard one. The eggs are counted in the entire preparation and counts are expressed per direct smear or per amount of faeces. In general smears prepared from experienced technician contain not less than 1mg or more than 2mg of formed faeces.

Dilution Egg Counts

Fill the flask upto 56ml mark with 0.4% N/10 NaOH and add faeces to bring the contents up to 60ml mark. Add beads to the flask and shake vigorously. Allow it to stand for 12-24 hours with occasional shaking. Take out exactly 0.075ml from the flask and put it on a slide. Cover it with cover glass and systematically count all eggs present. Multiply the count with 200 that records count as eggs per gram of faeces. However, to arrive at a correct number of eggs, the figure is multiplied by 1 for hard, difficult to puncture faeces, by 2 for mushy formed faeces that can be cut by applicator, by 3 for mushy diarrheic faeces taking shape of container and by 4 for diarrheic but not watery faeces where as watery faeces are not suitable for egg counts.

It has been shown that egg counts made from direct smear samples are as reliable as those made by dilution methods. The egg counts are only rough estimates of egg out put because of the fact that the eggs are not evenly distributed in the faeces and eggs contributed to the faeces by worms in small and large intestine are eliminated over a period of 1 to 7 days as a result of reflex of contents of the caecum and upper colon.

Fluorescent Antibody Test (FAT)

This test is used for the diagnosis of many infectious bacterial or viral diseases and is having outstanding advantage of detecting antigen while still in tissues, cells or specimens, even after fixation. However, it requires fluorescence microscope that is expensive. This technique involves attaching of a fluorescent labeled antibody on viral or bacterial antigens within the cells, tissues, smears or cell cultures. Antigen and antibody detection is explored by observing fluorescence given by fluorescent dye labeled antibody. However, in negative tests no fluorescence is observed because the dye labeled antibody gets washed down if not fixed to antigen.

This test can be performed directly by allowing labeled antibody to fix with antigen or indirectly by allowing antibody antigen fixation and thereafter allowing second fluorescent labeled antibody (anti antibody) to fix itself with primary antibody forming a complex with antigen and can be observed with fluorescent microscope. The test can best be understood from given flowchart.

Haemagglutination Test (HA)

Certain viruses belonging to the influenza group like Myxoviruses, Togaviruses, Reoviruses, some Adenoviruses and Poxviruses agglutinate the washed red blood cells of various species of animals and is called haemagglutination. Viruses attach

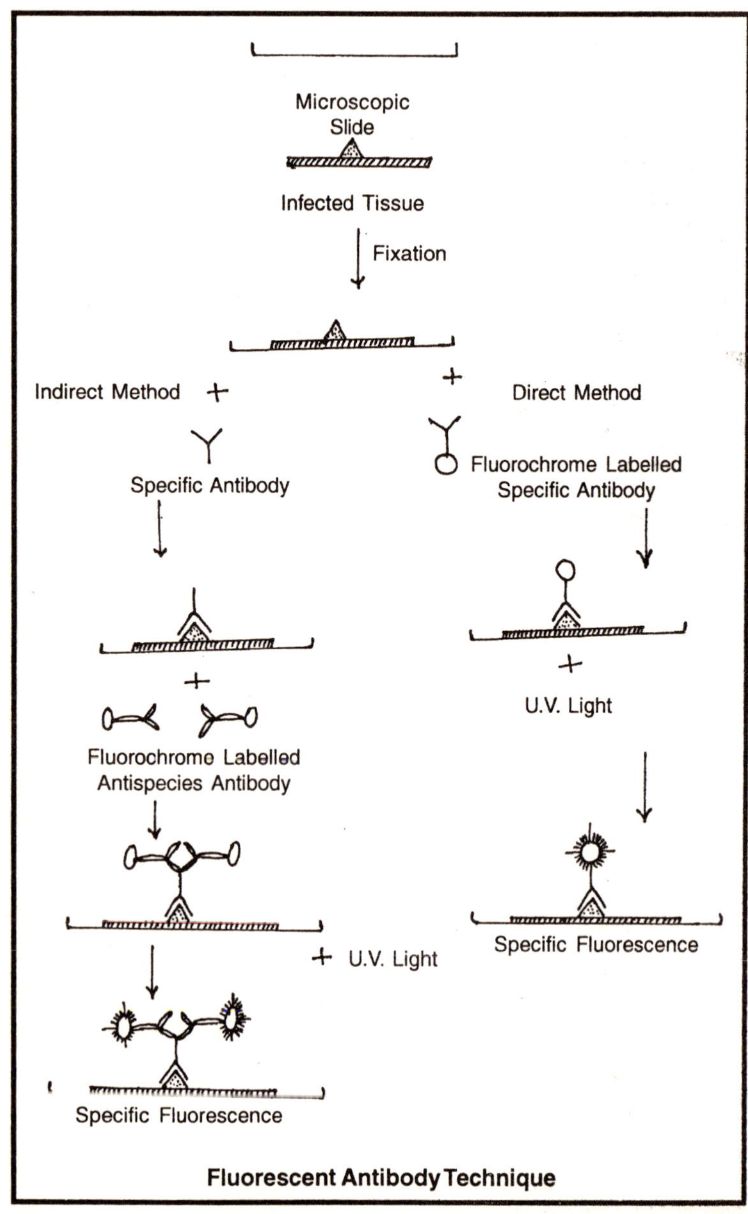

Fluorescent Antibody Technique

themselves to the surface of red blood cells by means of enzymatic groups reacting with mucopolysaccharide substrate of red cells, in exactly the same way as they adhere to the surface of epithelial cells of the bronchioles, causing agglutination of red cells. Red cells fall rapidly in the suspended fluid to settle on the bottom in an irregular ragged pattern instead forming button on the bottom in the control test.

It is an important, simple and rapid method of detecting virus in egg or tissue culture fluids, besides provides a basis for purification of virus.

Procedure

1. Take a clean, clear microtitre plate having 96 (8 rows and 12 columns) U shaped wells.
2. Place 50µl of normal saline or phosphate buffer saline pH 7.2 into 12 wells of 1st row with the help of a micropipette.
3. Add 50µl of suspected viral fluid in the first well and mix thoroughly and gently by drawing the fluid in the pipette several times.(dilution 1:1)
4. Take 50µl from 1st well and add it to 2nd well, mix the two and take 50ul from 2nd well to 3rd well (dilution 1:4). Continue the process of serial dilution of suspected material until well 11th (dilution 1:1032) and from 11th well discard 50µl.
5. Well 12th serves as control with no suspected material.
6. Add 50µl of 1% RBC suspension (saline or PBS washed fowl red blood cells) to each well from 1st to 12th.
7. Shake the plate gently and carefully by agitating, with out spelling out contents from the wells.
8. Incubate the plate at room temperature and read the test at intervals of 15, 20, 30, 45 minutes.
9. Observe the control well for sedimentation of red cells as a button at the bottom. If the sedimentation is not found repeat the test.
10. Presence of virus and its concentration is determined by the agglutination of red cells which will not sediment at the bottom of a well but shall form a layer of uniformly agglutinated cells covering the bottom of wells

11. The virus titre is expressed as HA units contained in undiluted sample or reciprocal of the end point dilution.

Haemagglutination Inhibition Test (HI)

When the viruses which produce haemagglutination of red cells are charged with antibodies against the virus, results in the loss of ability of virus to cause haemagglutination. This test is successfully employed for identifying new virus isolates and for the determination of antibody titres to HA antigens.

Procedure

1. Determine the H.A titre of the stock virus as described under HA test..
2. Divide HA titre by 4 to make 4 HAU antigen.(if HA titre is 1:320, 4 HAU will be 1:80 i.e. 1 part of antigen is diluted with 80 parts of diluent).
3. Position a clear, clean microtitre plate having 96 U shaped wells.
4. Place 50µl of phosphate buffer saline in 12 wells of first and second row.
5. Add 50µl of normal serum (heat inactivated at 56^{0}C for 30 minutes) to first well of first row. Mix the serum and PBS thoroughly with the help of pipette and then transfer 50µl to 2nd well of first row and make serial dilution of the serum in first row till 12th well is reached and discard 50µl from the 12th well.
6. Add 50µl of test serum/antiserum (heat inactivated) in the 1st well of second row, mix well and transfer 50µl to 2nd well and so on serially diluting the serum as in first row.
7. Add 50µl of virus antigen containing 4HAU to each well of first and second row.
8. Add 50µl of 1% washed RBCs to all wells.
9. Agitate the plate gently and carefully to ensure even suspension of RBCs in the mixture.
10. Incubate the test plate at room temperature and read after 15 to 30 minutes or until clear haemagglutination has appeared.
11. Examine the first row for haemagglutination and if it is not there repeat the test.

12. Test serum containing HI antibodies will inhibit the agglutination of cells in second row and HI titre is expressed as reciprocal of the highest dilution of serum inhibiting agglutination. HI titre of 2^5 or more is considered positive.

Histopathology Technique

Histopathology technique involves many processes and are described as under.

Collection and Fixation

1. The materials should be collected immediately after death and taken from the portion representing characteristic lesion.
2. For micro-anatomical studies the material should be kept in 10% formal saline (100ml formaldehyde + 900 ml distilled water + 8.5 g sodium chloride) and for cytology the fixatives used are Flemming's fluid (Chromic acid 15ml + 2% osmic acid 4 ml + glacial acetic acid 1ml) or Carony's fluid (absolute alcohol 60ml +chloroform 30ml + glacial acetic acid 10ml).
3. The fixative should be ten to twenty times more than the volume of the tissue.

Washing

1. Keep the tissue under running water for 12 hours. Ellis histopathological tank can be used for this purpose.

Dehydration

1. After thorough washing, the tissues are dehydrated by passing them in ascending grades through a series of bottles having different percentage of alcohol.
2. The serial dipping of tissue in ascending grades of alcohol prevents sudden fold like appearance of the tissue.
3. Alcohol 30% for 30 minutes.
4. Alcohol 50% for 30 minutes.
5. Alcohol 70% for 30 minutes.
6. Alcohol 90% for 30 minutes.
7. Absolute alcohol No.I for 30 minutes.
8. Absolute alcohol No.II for 6 hours.

Clearing

1. Clearing of the tissue is done by dipping the tissue in Xylol No.I for 30 min. or Cedar wood oil for 30 min.
2. Then dipping is performed in Xylol No. II for 2 to 6 hours or cedar wood oil No. II till it becomes clear.

Paraffin Embedding

1. After clearing, the tissue is dipped in the melted paraffin in paraffin oven that maintains its melting point.
2. The tissue is dipped in four serially arranged buckets with melted paraffin keeping in each bucket for one hour and for 4 hrs in last bucket.
3. The "L" mould made either of brass or glass is put on the brass plate and is made rectangular by two L moulds in which melted paraffin is poured.
4. Tissue is kept in the middle of melted paraffin and a heated forcep is allowed to go round the tissue once to expel the air.
5. Paraffin block is available after removing the "L" moulds.
6. The blocks are kept in a cool place for easy and good cutting.

Cutting and Mounting

1. Heat the block holder and attach the holder with the paraffin block and keep it in a cool place for 5 minutes.
2. Fit the block fitted holder to the microtome machine.
3. Adjust the thickness of the section between 4-6 microns.
4. Cut the sections by revolving the wheel of machine.
5. Lift the cutting tissue sections with the help of section lifter and put it in the enameled dish containing hot water heated to 45°c to spread it.
6. Take the slides and smear with Mayer's glycerin egg albumin (1 gm sod.salicylate + 50ml glycerol + 50 ml of egg albumin, mix and filter).
7. Place the cut sections from the hot water over the slide.
8. Stain the sections as described.

Staining of the Mounted Sections by Haematoxylin and Eosin Stain

1. Deparaffinisation is done by dipping the mounted tissue sections into;

   (a) Xylol No.I for 5 minutes

   (b) Xylol No.II for 5 minutes.

2. Before staining, the tissue is to be brought to water level by passing it through;

   (a) 90% alcohol for 3-5 minutes

   (b) 70% alcohol for 3-5 minutes

   (c) 30% alcohol for 3-5 minutes

   (d) The slide is then kept in distilled water for 5 minutes and thus tissue comes to water level.

3. Keep the sections in a jar containing Haematoxylin stain for 5 minutes staining the nucleus violet in colour.
4. Remove the excess stain by putting the sections in acid alcohol for 1 minute.
5. Wash the sections by dipping in distilled water 3-4 times.
6. Bleach the sections by dipping in Ammonia water and then again in distilled water.
7. Stain the sections with eosin for 5 minutes to colour the cytoplasm reddish pink.
8. Wash the sections with distilled water.
9. Dehydrate it to remove the water by passing it through;

   (a) 30% alcohol for 5 minutes

   (b) 50% alcohol for 5 minutes

   (c) 70% alcohol for 5 minutes

   (d) 90% alcohol for 5 minutes

   (e) absolute alcohol No.I for 5 minutes and

   (f) absolute alcohol No.II for 5 minutes

10. Keep the sections in jars containing;

    (a) Xylol No.I and

    (b) Xylol No.II for 5 minutes

11. Finally mount the sections with cover slips by Canada Balsum or DPX and examine the slides under microscope for histopathology.

Note

Freezing technique is used to get results within half an hour or for special studies of tissue structure, while avoiding use of preservatives, alcohol, xylol etc. Carbon dioxide is used to freeze the tissue and harden it to cut the freezed tissue by freezing microtome in very short time. There after paraffin embedding is proceeded.

Inoculation Techniques

Animal inoculation tests are of great importance in isolation of organisms from mixed cultures, evaluation of quality of vaccines, pharmaceutical products, passaging and maintenance of seed culture and in the animal disease diagnosis.

In all cases the animal to be inoculated should be restrained and held firmly in easy position. The site of inoculation must be prepared by shaving or clipping of hairs, cleansing of the area by alcohol (70%) or betadine besides keeping all the necessary things in readiness. The syringe and needles used for inoculation should be sterile. Animal inoculation is performed by various routes depending upon the test and material employed.

Intradermal Inoculation

It is better to select white animals or white areas if skin reactions are to be elicited like allergy tests, Tuberculin, Jhonin tests.

1. Prepare the inoculation site (skin of neck in large animals, abdomen in laboratory animals) as discussed above.
2. A sterilized 1ml syringe with 26-gauge needle is inserted in a pinched-up fold of skin as superficially as possible.
3. Successful inoculation is evidenced with the development of a raised white anaemic spot.
4. Intradermal inoculation in rabbit and guinea pig requires practice owing to their thin skins.
5. The amount injected intradermally should not exceed 0.01ml.

Subcutaneous Inoculation

1. Inoculations are generally performed in the median line of the abdominal wall or in the groin or neck after the preparation of the site.
2. Pinch-up a fold of skin between forefinger and thumb of the left hand with a syringe in right hand.
3. Insert the needle into the ridge of skin between finger and thumb and push steadily onward till needle is inserted about an inch.
4. Relax the grasp of left hand and slowly inject the material.
5. If skin gets raised it indicates success of inoculation.

However, if solid material is to be injected subcutaneously, it is deposited by giving an incision through the skin. The skin is then separated from underlying muscles and a pocket is formed and the material is deposited in the pocket as far as possible from the point of entrance. Closure of the wound may require a stitch.

Intramuscular inoculation:

1. Inoculations are usually made in the posterior muscles of thigh or lateral thoracic or abdominal muscles.
2. Prepare the site of inoculation.
3. Steady the skin over the selected muscles with the slightly separated left forefinger and thumb.
4. Thrust the needle into the muscular tissue quickly.
5. Before the material is deposited in the tissue draw the piston of syringe back to ensure that needle is not in a blood vessel and then slowly inject the inoculum.

Intravenous Inoculation

Intravenous inoculation requires identification of vein to be inoculated which is facilitated by applying pressure on the vein in the opposite direction of its flow and vein is raised which can be easily felt.

The intravenous inoculation is carried in different veins in different animals. In cattle, sheep, goat and horses it is best to inoculate jugular vein at the base of neck. In rabbits it is the posterior auricular vein along the outer margin of ear. In guinea pigs large superficial veins lying on the dorsal and inner aspect of hind leg are well suited for intravenous inoculation. In mice lateral veins of the tail running parallel to the tail are best adopted for intravenous inoculation

1. The needle is inserted through the skin and wall of vein until it enters the lumen of vein.
2. Ensure the needle is in vein by drawing the piston of syringe back and if blood comes into syringe it confirms the needle in vein.
3. If blood does not come into the syringe, gently manipulate the needle under the skin to push it in the vein.
4. Slowly inject the inoculum.
5. Withdraw the needle quickly and apply a firm compression with the help of cotton swab at the puncture wound to arrest bleeding.

Intra-cardial Inoculation

Guinea pigs, mice and rabbits may be inoculated by intracardial route instead of intravenous. The technique is not more difficult and no ill effects have been observed.

1. The animal is tied to an operating board or held firmly by an assistant.
2. Sometimes anesthetics may be given.
3. The point of maximum pulsation to the left of the sternum by palpation is determined and the site is prepared for inoculation.
4. A sharp thin long needle is inserted at the selected point.
5. A rush of blood in the syringe indicates the success of technique.
6. Slowly inject the inoculum.

Intra-abdominal or Intra-peritoneal Inoculation

1. The inoculation area in the median abdominal line, just below umbilicus, is shaved and cleaned with 2% iodine in alcohol.

2. Animal is held firmly upon its back with abdomen facing operator.
3. Syringe is grasped firmly and needle inserted through the skin for a short distance in the direction of head in the long axis of animal, the hand is then raised and needle forced forward through peritoneum which is evidenced by the relaxation of abdominal muscles.
4. The needle is slightly withdrawn and inoculum deposited.
5. It can also be performed by pinching up the entire thickness of abdominal parieties in a fold and slip the peritoneal surfaces over each other to ascertain that no intestinal loops are included.
6. Insert the needle at the base of the fold.
7. Release the fold and inoculate.
8. Any swelling at the inoculation indicates needle in subcutaneous tissue and an attempt be made to enter the peritoneum.

Johnin Test

This is not sufficiently dependable diagnostic test, yet it is significantly accurate.

Procedure

1. Clip, shave and cleanse with alcohol an area of 6 inches in the middle of neck.
2. Grasp the skin in the middle of prepared area tightly with the help of thumb and forefinger and measure the thickness of skin with the use of caliper.
3. Inject 0.1ml of johnin intradermally by a tuberculin syringe.
4. Take the reaction reading after 48 hours.
5. In positive cases there is painful edematous swelling or thickness of skin increased by 4mm or more.
6. In negative case no swelling is displayed.

Intravenous Johnin Test

1. It is claimed to be more reliable test than intradermal.
2. Inject 2ml of Johnin in jugular vein.

3. Increase in rectal temperature by 1.5 °F, within 6 to 8 hours, indicates positive reaction.

Mallein Test

1. It is an intradermo-palpebral test used as a diagnostic test in glanders (actinobacillosis).
2. 0.1 to 0.2ml of mallein, supplied by IVRI, is injected intradermally in the lower eyelid with the use of tuberculin syringe.
3. The readings are taken after 24 to 48 hours.
4. In positive cases there is marked edema of eyelid with blephero-spasm and sever purulent conjunctivitis.

Mastitis Test

Bromothymol Blue Test

In mastitis the pH of milk changes from normal acidic to alkaline which can be detected by bromothymol blue test.

1. Take 1ml of bromothymol blue solution (1g bromothymol blue dissolved in 160ml N/100 NaOH + 590ml distilled water) in a graduated tube.
2. Add to it 5ml of freshly drawn milk.
3. Mix the two gently.
4. Development of green or blue colour indicates presence of inflammatory exudates in milk, hence positive for mastitis.

Chloride Test

This test can be easily performed and is based on the principle that in mastitis chloride content of milk gets increased.

1. Take 1ml of fresh milk in a test tube add to it 5ml of silver nitrate solution (0.134% aq solution).
2. Add to it two drops of 10% potassium chromate solution and mix.
3. Observe for yellow colour in positive mastitis cases.

Drug Sensitivity Test (Antibiogram)

The test is of paramount importance in clinical medicine for effective treatment of diseases. Bacterial or fungal infections are better to be treated after performing drug sensitivity test of the causative agent that helps in restraining the drug resistance being exhibited by the microbes. The test involves the subjection of causative agent/ agents to the effects of various antimicrobial drugs in in-vitro conditions to choose the better drug against the causative agent/ agents. The test is also performed to know the efficacy of different antimicrobial drugs/agents against known organism in-vitro. While performing this test the causative agent is first isolated, identified and subjected to drug sensitivity test. In cases of urgency, the test sample as such is subjected to drug sensitivity test with out any prior culture and isolation of organism from it. Through this test clinicians are able to know the best antimicrobial agent against the particular disease within hours. We have a wide range of antimicrobial discs available in the market now.

Procedure

1. Culture and isolate the causative organisms in a suitable medium.
2. Identify the organism and subculture it in a liquid medium.
3. Pour about 1ml of the broth, with good growth, on a blood agar or nutrient agar plate and allow it to spread all over the plate that can be facilitated by gentle to and fro agitation of plate or smearing on plate with the help of sterile swab or loop.
4. In case of quick assessment of effective drugs, spread or smear the sample as a whole (like milk, body fluids) over the plate.
5. Position the antimicrobial discs with the help of sterile forceps or disc dispensers on the agar.
6. Keep a suitable uniform distance between the discs.
7. Incubate the plate at 37°C for 6 -12 hours or even more.
8. After incubation, examine the plates for presence of growth and zone of inhibition around the discs.
9. Zone of inhibition around a disc suggests the sensitivity of organism against that drug and growth around the disc indicates the resistance of organism against that drug.
10. Depending upon the diameter of zone of inhibition, an organism is said to be highly, moderately or slightly susceptible to the drug. Roughly if zone of inhibition is more

than 25mm, it is highly susceptible, 10-20mm- moderately susceptible and less than 10mm slightly susceptible.

Milk Ring Test for Brucellosis

The antigen is supplied by Indian Veterinary Institute, Izatnagar. It is used to test the pooled bovine milk samples or individual samples from goat, sheep for detection of Brucellosis.

Procedure

1. Take 2ml of pooled milk (milk from 2 – 5 cows) in a tube.
2. Add two drops of antigen in the milk.
3. Shake the mixture by rotating between palms for a minute.
4. Incubate the mixture at 37°C for an hour.
5. After incubation place the tube at room temperature for 90 minutes.
6. Cherry coloured ring at the cream layer confirms the test positive for brucellosis.

Negri Body Detection

The definitive diagnosis of rabies does lie in the demonstration of intra-cytoplasmic Negri bodies, in the nerve cells of suspected animals.

Procedure

1. Negri bodies can be found in any portion of brain with nerve cells but are most numerous and characteristic in Ammon's horn or hippocampus.
2. Taking all precautionary measures, remove the brain of the animal.
3. Prepare simple contact smears of Ammon's horn by pressing clean, clear glass slide against the cut surface of the horn several times to allow the tissue to spread out over the slide.
4. While the smear is still moist, immerse the slide in a coplin jar containing Seller's stain for few seconds.
5. Use of smears fixed with methyl alcohol are less satisfactory.
6. Wash the slide in tap water and dry in air.
7. Examine the ganglion cells for Negri bodies which appear oval or round and bright cherry red in colour with basophilic

inner structures. Cytoplasm of cell stains blue to purplish blue, stroma are rose pink and neural sheaths unstained.

8. Inclusion bodies of distemper in dogs are pale pink, refractile and with out inner structures.
9. Examination of brain tissue sections is advisable if the direct smears are negative for Negri bodies.

Neutralization Test

Specific antibodies for a virus neutralize its infectivity and when such treated virus is injected into a susceptible host it does not produce infection. The amount of antibody present in the serum can be determined by this procedure, since higher the antibody titre, more will be the viruses neutralized. This test can be employed to test or identify an unknown serum or an unknown virus. If known virus is mixed with unknown serum, neutralization of infectivity identifies the antibodies in the test serum or if known serum is mixed with unknown virus, neutralization identifies the unknown virus. However this test may not be confirmatory when the two viruses have similar antigenic components.

This test is useful for titration of viral antibodies and in certain viral infections it is the only procedure available. This test requires living virus with determined activity and susceptible host cells such as chick embryos or tissue cultures.

Procedure

1. Serum is obtained from sick/ suspected/ recovered animal which serves as test serum and known antiserum serves as control.
2. Sera are heat inactivated at 56^{0}C for 30 minutes.
3. 1.5% of glucose or sucrose is added to the sera to prevent inhibitory factors.
4. Serial dilution of known virus is made in normal saline.
5. 50μl of each virus dilution is mixed with 50μl of saline and inoculated into each of 4 to 6 of 9-11 days old chick embryos via described routes for every disease (refer chapter 5 section-II)
6. 50μl of each virus dilution is mixed with 50μl of test serum and this mixture is allowed to stand for 15 – 30 minutes.

7. Inoculate this mixture of test serum and virus into each of 4 to 6 embryos.
8. Incubation of eggs is carried as in routine and examination of embryos by candling is done every day for any mortality and a record is kept for each dilution of both groups.
9. The dilution of virus as well as virus + serum which causes 50% mortality is recorded (50% end point).
10. The results are interpreted as :

Log of Neutralization index = – tive log of control titre — – tive log of virus + serum

Neutralization Index = anti log of figure obtained.

Example

Say 50% end point of virus dilution is 10^{-7} and 50% end point of virus + serum dilution is 10^{-3}, the log of neutralization index of serum = 7 – 3 = 4 (reciprocal of log). The capacity of serum to neutralize virus = 10^{-4} i.e. 10,000 times neutralizing antibodies are present in serum.

In cell cultures the end point is 50% reduction in the number of plaques in a fixed area of monolayer of cells instead of 50% mortality in embryo culture.

Polyacrylamide Gel Electophoresis (PAGE)

The technique is employed in the analysis of proteins, ribosomal proteins, histones etc. thereby plays a major role in the analysis, diagnosis and confirmation of various antigenic agents. The technique is based on the principle that any charged ion or group will migrate towards electrodes when placed in an electric field. Electrophoresis of any protein mixture will result in migration of different proteins at different rates towards one of the electrodes and proteins of different mobilities travel as discrete zones which gradually separate from each other as the process of electrophoresis proceeds. Electrophoresis is carried out in a solution stabilized within a supporting medium like sheets of paper, silica gel, alumina or cellulose which are spread as a thin layer on glass or plastic plates and gels of agarose starch or polyacrylamide. The starch and polyacrylamide gels are porous and the pore size is of the same order as the size of protein molecule so that a sieving effect occurs and the separation becomes both charge density and size dependent.

This type of electrophoresis is of great importance in identifying the two proteins of different sizes but identical charge densities.

Polyacrylamide gel is a synthetic polymer of acrylamide monomer, transparent, chemically inert and stable over a wide range of pH, temperature and ionic strength and best suited for electrophoresis of most proteins. Flat slab gels of 0.75 – 1.5mm thick are preferred over cylindrical tube gels because many samples including molecular mass marker proteins can also be electrophoresed under identical conditions in a single gel such that the band patterns produced are directly comparable. Slab gels allow densitometry, photography and can easily be dried for storage or autoradiography.

PAGE of proteins use a buffer system designed to dissociate all proteins into their individual polypeptides. Most commonly dissociating agent used is the ionic detergent, Sodium Dodecyl Sulphate (SDS) and typical buffer system used are Tris-glycine (pH 8.3-9.5), Tris-borate (pH 8.3-9.3), Tris-acetate (pH 7.2-8.5) and Tris-citrate(pH 7-8.5). About 90% of complex protein mixtures, even crude cell lysates, will enter the gel if SDS is the dissociating agent.

Protein mixture is denatured by heating at 100°C in presence of excess SDS and a thiol reagent (2-mercaptoethanol or dithiothreitol) to cleave disulphide bands. Most polypeptides bind SDS in a constant weight ratio (1.4g of SDS per gram of polypeptide). PAGE, besides analyzing the polypeptide composition of the sample, can determine the molecular mass of the polypeptides by reference to the mobility of polypeptides of known molecular mass under same electrophoretic conditions. PAGE can be carried out at a pH anywhere between 3 and 10. Nucleic acids can be removed by selective extraction or precipitation procedures. Histones can be acid extracted from chromatin, RNA of ribosomes is precipitated with HCl leaving the proteins in solution or high molecular weight nucleic acids are removed by ultracentrifugation at 100000g for 24 hours at 5°C in which pellets formed are RNA where as DNA band in the bottom half of the gradient and protein concentrated at the top of gradient.

Apparatus Required

1. Gel holders and electrophoresis panels
2. 15 W day light fluorescent lamp for photo-polymerisation of

riboflavin catalyzed polyacrylamide gel.

3. Micropipette or micro-liter syringes for loading of sample on to gel.
4. A peristaltic pump for preparation of acrylamide concentration gradient gel and for over-layering of all slab gels to obtain a flat gel surface.
5. Power pack capable of supplying about 500v and 100mA

Points to be Adopted in PAGE

1. About 1-10µg of each polypeptide and 50-100µg for a complex mixture is usually sufficient to be loaded on to gel. Overloading or under loading of sample results in distorted bands and minor components are not detected. Best results are obtained with the use of sample volumes of 10 to 30µl.
2. Best results are obtained with use of 1.5mm thick slab gel and 7mm wide wells.
3. It is important to have SDS present in excess atleast 5% SDS can be added without deleterious effects.
4. Prior to electrophoresis and immediately after the addition of SDS, samples are heated in a boiling water bath for 3 minutes to ensure denaturation of protein and then allowed to cool at room temperature.
5. Any insoluble material should be removed by centrifugation (12000g for 5 minutes).
6. The sample may be used immediately or stored in the freezer at -20°C and should be warmed before use.
7. It is desirable to pre-electrophorese the gel for a period of 30-40 minutes prior to loading the sample.
8. It is good to add a marker (bromophenol blue) to the sample to mark the progress of electrophoresis.
9. The recommended running conditions at a constant current of 20mA is 4 hours.

Staining of Gels

Protein bands of sufficiently high concentration may be demonstrated by direct photometric scanning of unstained gels at 280nm. However, the usual method is to increase the sensitivity of protein detection by reacting the protein bands with an easily visualized reagent/ stain.

Silver staining is the most sensitive staining.

1. It is important to remove the substances like buffers, detergents or reducing agents which may interfere with the staining and then only silver staining is allowed.
2. The gel is exposed to silver nitrate solution and reduction of silver nitrate to metallic silver at a protein band with the deposition of silver grains on it, is the basic mechanism involved in this staining.
3. To ensure the good circulation of staining solution around the gel, it is better to keep the gel tray on platform shaker.

Radio-labeling

The major advantage of radio-labeling is that the radiolabelled proteins following gel electophoresis are far more sensitive than staining methods for unlabelled proteins. This technique of radio-labeling is approached either by placing the gel next to the X-ray film where upon the radioactive emissions cause the production of silver atoms within silver halide crystals and are visualized after developing the film or slicing of gel after electrophoresis and determining the radioactive content of each slice which is most commonly used for quantification of radioactive proteins.

Radioimmunoassay

It is developed as a result of combination of immunological and radionuclide techniques and is extremely sensitive assay technique. Substances of physiological and pharmaceutical importance are readily assayed by this technique even in levels down to picogram. This technique is useful in assaying the substances which are incapable of direct measurement such as hormones, peptides, cyclic AMP, prostaglandins etc.

The technique is based on the principle of isotope dilution and depends on the availability of specific antibody to the measuring substance and availability of that substance in radio labeled form. The test can detect the unknown antigen or unknown antibody by radio-immunoprecipitation. It involves fixing of known antigen or antibody to polypropylene microwells. The test is rapid, sensitive and specific. It can be best understood from the given flow chart.

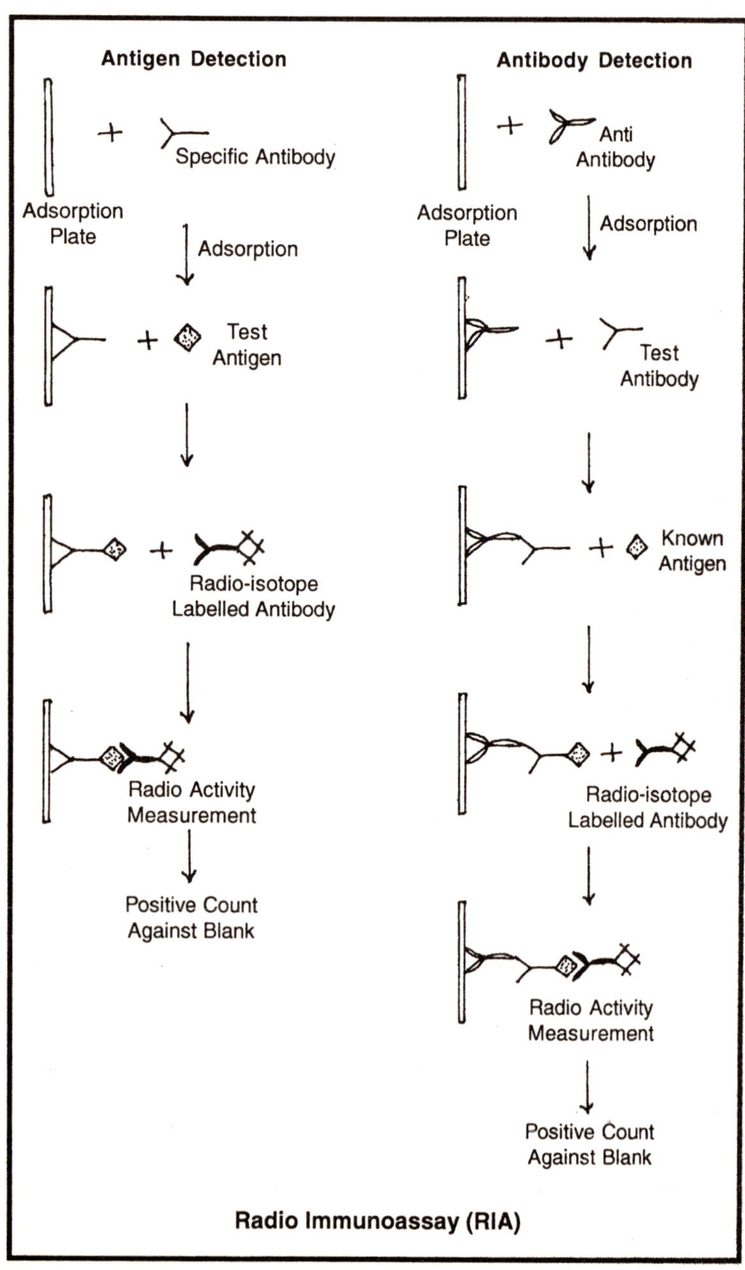

Radio Immunoassay (RIA)

Rapid Test for Brucellosis with Coloured Antigen

1. Coloured brucella antigen is supplied by IVRI and is used to detect the brucella infection in the animals from its serum sample.
2. Pour 0.08ml or two drops and 0.04ml or one drop of test serum at the two ends of a clean glass slide.
3. Add a drop of coloured antigen in the vicinity of the test serum at two ends of slide and mix the two gently with the help of a pin or stick.
4. Ensure proper mixing by rotating the slide.
5. In positive cases there is aggregation of antigen in clumps in 4 to 5 minute.
6. In negative cases there is no flocculation.
7. If the clumping is only in 0.08ml serum spot, the test is claimed suspicious and should be confirmed by tube agglutination test.

Rapid Test for Pullorum with Coloured Antigen

1. Place a loopful of whole blood on the glass plate.
2. Add a drop of coloured antigen in the close vicinity of blood drop.
3. Mix the two with the help of stick and by tilting the plate.
4. In positive cases there is clumping of red cells and floating in clear fluid within a minute.
5. Delayed reaction is claimed to be suspicious and should be confirmed by tube test.

Rose Bengal Plate Agglutination Test for Brucellosis

This test is similar to the rapid plate test with coloured antigen. The difference is in the staining of antigen. In this test the antigen is stained with rose Bengal stain. It is supplied from Veterinary Biologicals, Banglore.

Procedure

1. Pour 0.08ml or two drops and 0.04ml or one drop of test serum at the two ends of a clean glass slide.
2. Add a drop of Rose Bengal antigen in the vicinity of the test

serum at two ends of slide and mix the two gently with the help of a pin or stick.

3. Ensure proper mixing by rotating the slide.
4. In positive cases there is aggregation of antigen in clumps in 4 to 5 minutes.
5. In negative cases there is no flocculation.
6. If the clumping is only in 0.08ml serum spot, the test is claimed suspicious and should be confirmed by tube agglutination test.

Tuberculin Test/Montoux Test

Tuberculin is an extract containing specific protein of Tubercle bacilli and the test is based on exhibition of tissue hypersensitivity. The test is being used in man and animals to detect the presence of tuberculosis in active or latent form.

In animals tuberculin from Indian Veterinary Research Institute is used as intradermal injection in the neck region at 0.1ml dose.

Procedure

1. Clip, shave and cleanse with alcohol an area of 6 inches in the middle of neck.
2. Grasp the skin in the middle of prepared area tightly with the help of thumb and forefinger and measure the thickness of skin with the use of caliper.
3. Inject 0.1ml of tuberculin intradermally by a tuberculin syringe.
4. Take the reaction reading after 48 hours.
5. In positive cases there is painful swelling or thickness of skin gets increased by 4mm or more.
6. In case no defined edema is recorded except a button is present, inject 0.1ml of tuberculin at the first site of injection and take the readings at 72 hours interval.
7. Positive cases shall have hot, painful and edematous swelling where as negative cases do not display any swelling.

In birds tuberculin 0.2ml is injected into one wattle, where as second wattle serves as control. In positive cases there will be hot, painful and edematous swelling in 48 hours.

Short Thermal Tuberculin Test

1. 4ml tuberculin is injected subcutaneously in the neck of the animal with rectal temperature not more than 102^{0}F.
2. Positive reactors have elevated rectal temperature, above 104^{0}F in 4 to 8 hours duration.
3. It is generally employed in the animals with negative intradermal test. This test is performed with caution because deaths do occur due to anaphylaxis reaction.

Tube Agglutination Test for Brucellosis

Brucella plain antigen is supplied by Indian Veterinary Institute, Izatnagar.

Procedure

1. Take 5 agglutination tubes in a rack.
2. Put 0.8ml of saline in first tube and 0.5ml in rest of the tubes.
3. Add 0.2ml of test serum into the 1st tube i.e. 1:5 dilution and mix thoroughly.
4. Transfer 0.5ml from 1st tube to the 2nd (1:10) and from 2nd to the 3rd tube and so on serially till last tube, only after thorough mixing in each dilution.
5. Discard 0.5ml from last tube. Add 0.5ml of plain antigen in each tube and mix well. Now each tube contains 1ml of serum antigen mixture.
6. A tube with 0.5ml saline and 0.5ml antigen serves as control.
7. Incubate the tubes in a bacteriological incubator at 37^{0}C for 24 hours.
8. After taking out from the incubator, keep the test tubes at atmospheric temperature for an hour and then take readings.
9. The positive tubes will be clear, transparent with no turbidity where as negative tubes will have turbidity.
10. Agglutination in the first 3 tubes indicates positive for brucellosis i.e. 1:40 dilution.

Tube Agglutination Test for Pullorum

The antigen for the test is supplied from Indian Veterinary Institute, Izatnagar.

Procedure

1. Take 5 agglutination tubes in a rack.
2. Put 0.8ml of saline in first tube and 0.5ml in rest of the tubes.
3. Add 0.2ml of test serum into the 1st tube i.e. 1:5 dilution and mix thoroughly.
4. Transfer 0.5ml from 1st tube to the 2nd (1:10) and from 2nd to the 3rd tube and so on serially till last tube, only after thorough mixing in each dilution.
5. Discard 0.5ml from last tube. Add 0.5ml of plain antigen in each tube and mix well. Now each tube contains 1ml of serum antigen mixture.
6. A tube with 0.5ml saline and 0.5ml antigen serves as control.
7. Incubate the tubes in a bacteriological incubator at 37^0C for 24 hours.
8. After taking out from the incubator, keep the test tubes at atmospheric temperature for an hour and then take the readings.
9. The positive tubes will be clear, transparent with no turbidity where as negative tubes will have turbidity.
10. Agglutination in the first 3 tubes indicates positive for brucellosis i.e. 1:40 dilution.

Thin Layer Immunoassay

This technique is used to detect the antigen antibody reaction. It is based on the principle of absorbing globulins as a thin layer on a polystyrene surface and such an antibody coated surface has the characteristics of an immuno-sorbant, able to bind the antigens. Antigen antibody reaction becomes visible when the surface is exposed to water vapour, because the surface on which antigen antibody reaction has taken place is hydrophilic and large water drops are formed in contrast to the background which is hydrophobic. The difference in the condensation patterns is easily recognized by the naked eye and does not require any sophisticated equipment. However the sensitivity of this method remains low. The test can best be understood in the given flow chart.

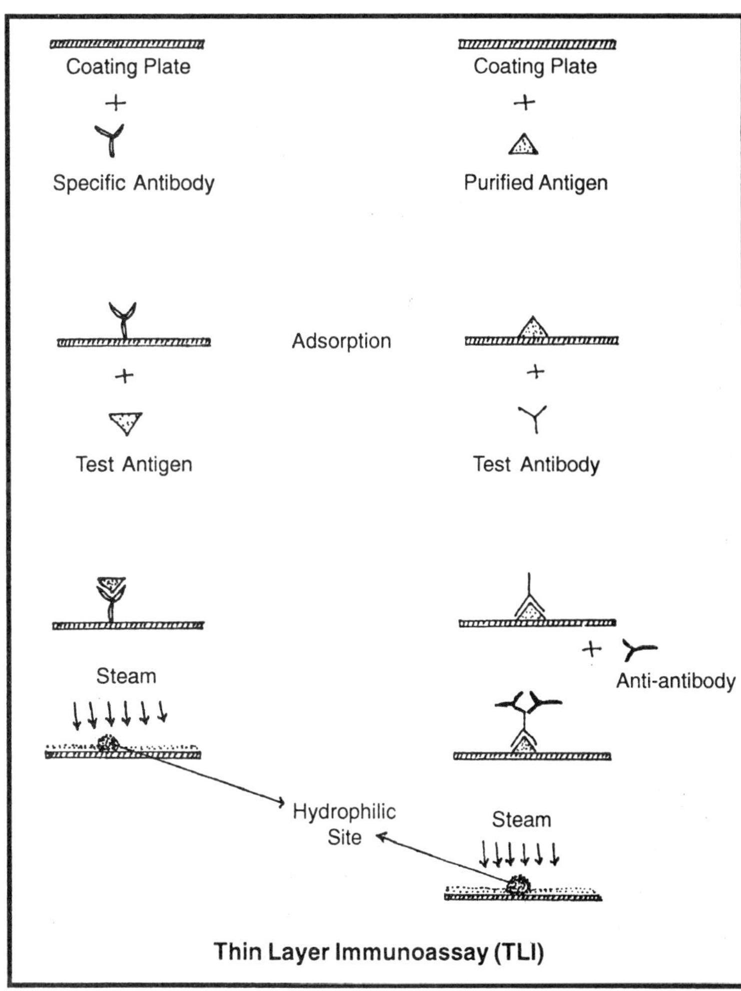

Thin Layer Immunoassay (TLI)

Chapter 7

Care and Management of Laboratory Animals

The laboratory animals are of paramount importance, not only in arriving at a disease diagnosis but also in evaluation of safety and potency of vaccines and pharmaceutical agents. It is important to maintain the well being and proper health of laboratory animals which demands high degree of skill and full understanding of their ways of life. Commonly used laboratory animals are discussed in detail here under.

Mice

Housing

The ideal home for mice has proved to be a wooden box of uniform size which can easily be taken for cleaning. However, to avoid the gnaw of their way out, aluminum sheets are used to cover the sides of the box. The lid of the box should have open area covered with perforated aluminum sheet to allow sufficient ventilation. It is better to have tray, bottom of which is covered with saw dust or wood shavings or news paper strips. However, now more comfortable plastic mice cages are available, having stainless steel lid provided with the facility for water bottle and feed. Boxes are cleaned at least twice a week and old bedding replaced by new.

Feeding

Feeding should be done in hoppers that may be suspended wire baskets inside the cage or depressed wire mesh containers incorporated into the lids of cages. A simple, safe and efficient arrangement to provide water is in an inverted glass bottle with glass or stainless steel nipples attached by means of a rubber cork or soft plastic cap. Pelleted mice feed is available and best suited for the mice. Fresh drinking water should be provided.

Handling

A grip should be taken at the middle of the tail by left hand and raising gently the hind limbs. Then with the right hand finger and thumb a fold of skin should be taken as closely to the head as possible. This way mouse can be restrained and lifted into a convenient position for laboratory procedures like inoculations.

Breeding

Male and female mice aged 8-12 weeks should be kept either in 1:1 ratio or 1:4 ratio in a cage. Where ratio is 1:1, there is no need to separate the pair and litters are produced after 3-4 weeks and the youngs should be weaned before the next litter is expected. However, where ratio is 1:4 the expected mouse should be separated, provided with a suitable soft bedding and allowed to nest and nurse her young until the age of three weeks.

Common Diseases

The common disease of mice include intestinal infections like Salmonellosis, septicemic disease like Pasteurellosis, Pseudotuberculosis caused by *Corynebacterium pseudotuberculosis*, Mouse septicaemia caused by Erysipelothrix., Mouse catarrh caused by PPLO. Some viral diseases are Mouse Pox, Lymphocyctic choriomeningitis and Encephalomyelitis.

Rabbits

Housing

Rabbit pens are best placed under lean-to shelters, run walls made of 1 inch, floors ½ inch, of 18 or heavy gauge wire netting. Individual cages are best made of galvanized iron and a minimum size of the cage should be 2 x 2 x 1 ½ feet. Young rabbits up to the age of 3 months can be housed together but not after that and sexes need to be separated.

Feeding

Animals should be fed ad lib and fresh drinking water provided continuously. Coccidiostat may be incorporated in the diet. Pelleted feed is preferred. Vegetables or greens should be included in the daily ration.

Handling

Smooth back the ears of the animal and then grasp the ears and loose skin at the back of neck firmly with one hand and place the other hand under the hind quarters and lift the animal gently. Never lift the rabbit by ears alone. While removing from the cage place the animal on non slippery surface.

Breeding

It is done in batches of six, either by individual matting or running six females with one male. Doe is taken into the buck's cage and not buck in doe's cage for matting. Artificial insemination has a lot to offer the commercial breeder. Young rabbits are weaned at 6 weeks age and does are rematted as soon as possible. This cycle continues with out a break.

Common Diseases

Some of the common diseases of the rabbit are Coccidiosis, Pseudotuberculosis, Snuffles, Rabbit Syphilis, Ear Canker and Myxomatosis.

Guinea-Pigs

Housing

Housing is provided in pens that must be dry and sufficiently ventilated. Must be free from rodents as may carry the infection of salmonella or pasturella to the guinea pigs. One square foot of space should be provided for each animal and not more than 25 animals should be placed in one pen. Galvanized iron cages are recommended that can be easily washed and sterilized. Adult guinea pigs will survive the winter in unheated houses, but breeding under such conditions is not certain. In order to have continuous breeding artificial heating has to be arranged during winter to maintain 55-60°F with adequate ventilation.

Feeding

Guinea pigs can be reared on mash of bran and oats or alternatively a more balanced pellet diet may be used which can be fed from hopper. In addition to mash or cereal, hay and green food particularly the leaves and stems of cabbage, cauliflower must be given. Root vegetables along with green foods can be given. Fresh drinking water must be provided in some form.

Handling

Animal should be handled by placing one hand across the back of the animal with the thumb behind shoulders and fingers well forwarded to the other side. Lift the animal gently and support its weight with the other hand placed under hind quarters.

Breeding

Female guinea pig should not be mated before 4 months of age where as boar is fertile at the age of 3 months. Three to six sows should run with one boar which is ideal. The sows are allowed to have their litters in the common pen with boar and other sows of the group. In this type of establishment, the sows are matted immediately after the litter so that pregnancy is started with out delay. However, in this system, losses in newborn young are more, owing to less parental care. However in the system where the sows are transferred to separate pens during advanced pregnancy newly born ones get better managemental and parental care but number of litters is reduced from 5 in first system to about 3 in this system of rearing. Any female that does not rear to weaning at least ten youngs per year should be discarded.

Common Diseases

Most of the deaths in the guinea pigs are due to infections. The important ones are respiratory infections due to pneumococcus, streptococcus and haemophilus species. These infections mostly occur in winter months, encouraged by over crowding, cold and deficient diet. The serious infections are caused by pasturella and salmonella groups.

Hamsters

Housing

It is a small friendly rodent, attractive and easy to handle. It is a nocturnal animal, spends most of the time asleep during the day and very active during the night. The cages therefore should be large enough to permit him exercise and designed in a manner which will prevent his escape but allow sufficient ventilation. Cages may be made of galvanized iron, wood, plywood and fine wire mesh. A convenient size cage for a female and her litter should be approximately 12 x 6 x 7 inches. Floors of cages should be given a liberal covering of soft wood sawdust. In general an animal should be provided with a floor area of 72-80 sq.inch. Hamsters do well in a warm dry atmosphere, with temperature of 68-72°F and relative humidity 45-50%.

Feeding

Puppy biscuit meal with a supplement of fresh green food has been used successfully. Hamsters drink very little water, should be supplied in bottles with drinking spouts. Commercially available pelleted diet for mice, rats or guinea pigs is satisfactory basic diet.

Breeding

Hamsters are mated when they are 8-9 weeks. The gestation period is 16-17 days with a litter of eight or ten. The doe is only ready to accept the buck during a short period of time, occurring once every 4-5 days. The doe is put into buck's cage. The animals may fight viciously and when this occurs doe is returned to her cage. Doe is also kept with buck for 7-10 days but very often the doe refuses to let the buck eat and spends lot of time fighting and infact the buck may soon become all skin and bone. Youngs can be weaned at 3 to 4 weeks.

Common Diseases

Hamsters are prone to intestinal infections like Salmonellosis, Respiratory infections, Pneumonia, Mange and Leishmaniasis.

Rat

For many years rat has made a valuable contribution to scientific research because of its being intelligent and somewhat docile rodent. The Specific pathogen free (SPF) rats are now considered for recent scientific work and shall replace the conventional rat.

Housing

Housing of rats can be convenient in cages, placed in racks suspended from the ceiling or fixed to the walls, by brackets, in concrete rooms with artificial lighting and heating systems besides being well ventilated. Cages of metal or plastic or wood or combination of these are conveniently used. Plastic cages have an advantage of being easily cleaned and sterilized. A female with her litter should be given floor area of at least 140 sq. inch. Bedding should be of sawdust, wood shavings or oat chaff /oat husks.

Feeding

Feeding should be done in hoppers that may be suspended wire baskets inside the cage or depressed wire mesh containers incorporated into the lids of cages. A simple, safe and efficient arrangement to provide water is in an inverted glass bottle with glass or stainless steel nipples attached by means of a rubber bung or soft plastic cap. A complete diet is provided either as a cubed or pelleted diet or as whole grains or mashes made of locally available ingredients.

Handling

Docile rats can be handled in the same way as guinea pigs but while handling vicious rats, operator should wear leather gloves.

Breeding

The females become sexually mature at about 50-60 days where as the mating should not be until rats are atleast 90 days old. 1:1 male-female ratio or 2 : 6 ratio should be followed conveniently. Pregnant female should be separated and allowed to nest and nurse the young until they attain 3-4 weeks age, thereafter resting for 2 weeks, females should be mated again.

Common Diseases

Some of the common diseases of the rats are listed as Salmonellosis, Pneumonia, Bronchopneumonia, Middle ear disease, Mange or rat scabies besides nutritional deficiencies.

Note

Physiological data of laboratory animals is available at Chapter 9.

Chapter 8

Production of Common Livestock and Poultry Vaccines

Vaccination involves a controlled exposure of an animal to killed or avirulant strain of pathogen in order to stimulate the immune system and prepare it to confront virulent organism. Vaccination may prevent disease but not necessarily by preventing infection. It has been learned from epidemiological studies that sub-clinical infection after effective vaccination often consolidates immunity. Under the influence of antigen the lymphocytes change dramatically, nucleus becomes derepressed, cell begins to divide and reproduce daughter cells of the same antigenic specificity. Each stimulated cell can form a clone of effector cells, each reacting with same antigen. However, very soon after antigen contact, some of the proliferating cells revert to quiescent small lymphocytes known as memory cells.

Eventually as the immune response declines, effector cells are no longer active and totally replaced by clones of small lymphocyte memory cells. Within a clone all the lymphocytic cells have the same antigenic specificity as the original one. Memory cells lose their virgin status through contact with antigen and in case of B lymphocytes, known to produce a changed effector function, different classes of Ig with same antigen binding specificity get augmented upon second contact with antigen.

Anthrax Live Spore Vaccine

Seed Culture

A virulent anthrax (Bacillus anthracis) spore vaccine strain is procured from *Indian Veterinary Research Institute, Izatnagar* as freeze dried. The seed is suspended in broth or 50% glycerin saline and held in refrigerator.

Culture Medium

Plain agar medium containing

1. Agar 3 - 3.5%
2. Peptone 1%
3. Beef extract 1%
4. Sodium Chloride 0.5%, and
5. pH adjusted to 7.4.

Procedure

1. Streak out the seed culture in a nutrient agar plate and incubate it for 24 to 48 hours.
2. Pick out the isolated colony and examine it for purity.
3. Transfer the isolated colony into nutrient broth and incubate it overnight.
4. Check the purity of the broth and if found pure, use it as primary seed culture for commercial production of vaccine.
5. Place 150ml of plain agar in each clean roux flask.
6. Autoclave the medium at 15lb for 30 minutes.
7. Place the flasks horizontally and allow the medium to form a uniform layer of agar in the flask.
8. Incubate the flasks overnight and select only the sterile flasks for vaccine production.
9. Inoculate the selected, sterile roux flasks with 3ml of primary seed culture, while observing strict sterile measures, preferably in a laminar flow.
10. Spread the inoculum over the agar surface by to and fro movement of the flask.
11. Seal the flasks properly with cotton plugs and aluminium foil.
12. Incubate the flasks at 37°C for 72 hours.
13. After incubation examine the growth in flasks for purity.
14. Flasks with pure growth of anthrax organisms are selected for collection of growth.
15. Add about 15ml of sterile normal saline in each of selected flasks along with weighed sterile glass beads.

16. Scrape the whole growth by shaking the flask to and fro along with beads.
17. Pour out the washings in weighed sterile containers.
18. Record the weight of washings alone.
19. Add equal amount (by weight) of sterile, pure glycerin (pH 7.2) in to the container containing washings.
20. Mix the contents and leave the glycerinated culture in a cool dark place for 21 days with shaking the mixture everyday for few minutes.
21. Inoculate sub-cutaneously 2 guinea pigs with 0.5ml and other 2 with 0.2ml of 15 days glycerinated culture diluted 1 - 2 times. No death should be there, however, local reaction may be observed.
22. After 21 days determine the concentration of spores in the mixture by serial dilution of the stock and subsequent inoculation of known quantity on to the plate, after incubation numbers of colonies determine the number of spores per that volume of inoculum.
23. Dilute the glycerinated stock culture with 50% glycerin saline to make the concentration of 1 to 1.5 million spore per ml of culture mixture.
24. Bottling, sealing and labeling are done as per the laboratory standards.

Quality Control Tests

1. Inoculate a healthy sheep and a goat with 10ml of 21 days stock glycerinated suspension.
2. Inoculate another healthy sheep and a goat with 5ml of stock suspension.
3. Inoculate a healthy sheep and a goat with suspension containing 1 million spores.
4. Observe the animals for 21 days. None should die of anthrax.
5. Challenge test is performed in vaccinated animals with 100 O.L.D of virulent anthrax spore along with unvaccinated healthy 2 sheep and goats serving as controls.
6. The control animals should die of anthrax and none of the vaccinated should succumb.

7. The tested vaccine is ready for field use with its shelf life about 9 months at refrigeration temperature.

Black Quarter Vaccine

Seed Culture

Seed culture for the black quarter vaccine consists of two species of clostridium, *Clostridium chauvei* (strain 49) and *Clostridium septicum* (strain 51). It is also procured from IVRI, Izatnagar and is maintained by animal passage. The organisms are examined microscopically and biochemically for purity.

Culture Medium

The culture medium required is anaerobic medium, consisting of;

1. Peptone- 1%
2. Beef extract- 1%
3. Yeast Extract-0.5%
4. Liver extract- 0.5%
5. Potassium hydrogen phosphate-0.4%
6. Sodium chloride-0.5%
7. Sodium thioglycolate- 0.1%
8. Dextrose- 0.5% to 1% and
9. pH adjusted to 8 - 8.4 by sodium hydroxide.

The medium is autoclaved at 15lb pressure for 45 minutes in 5-10 litres quantity or for 20 minutes in little quantity. However, dextrose is not autoclaved but tyndalized (described in Chapter-1) and added to the medium at the time of inoculation.

Procedure

1. Primary seed is prepared in quantities of 100ml anaerobic broth, inoculated with seed organism separately for two species. Incubation is carried at 37°C for 36-48 hours. The growth is examined for purity and the best ones retained as primary seed culture.
2. For commercial production of vaccine, the medium is dispensed in 5-10 litre solution bottles and autoclaved at 15lbs pressure for 45 minutes.

3. The medium is tested for its sterility by incubating it overnight and only sterile bottles are selected for inoculation.
4. 50ml primary culture is inoculated in each selected bottle separately for two species of organism in 50:50 ratio, observing strict asepsis preferably in a laminar flow.
5. Add the tyndalized dextrose to each bottle to a concentration of 0.5% in medium.
6. Plug and seal the bottles and incubate at 37°C for 72 hours.
7. After incubation the growth is examined for purity and bottles with sufficient and desirable growth are formalized.
8. Formalization is done by adding formalin to a concentration of 0.5% in the product i.e. 5ml formaline per litre of broth.
9. Shake well the product and leave overnight in a cool dark place.
10. Formalized product is tested for sterility by inoculating fresh medium with formalized growth and incubated for 24 to 48 hours. No growth in fresh medium confirms formalization.
11. Bottling is done while mixing growths of two organisms at 50:50 ratio along with phenyl mercuric nitrate at a concentration of 0.002%.
12. Sealing and labeling is done as per the laboratory standards.

Quality Control Tests

Sterility Test

1. It is performed to confirm the killing of organisms with formalin.
2. 3% of samples are taken randomly from the final product.
3. 0.5ml to 1ml of formalized vaccine is inoculated in fresh aerobic as well as anaerobic culture tubes.
4. Incubated for 24 to 72 hours.
5. After incubation if tubes exhibit growth, repeat the procedure while as no growth confirms the successful formalization and product as sterile.

Safety and Potency Test

1. Six guinea pigs are inoculated subcutaneously with 2-3ml of product.

2. If no death occurs within 5 days, vaccine is said to be safe.
3. After 14 days these vaccinated guinea pigs are grouped in two, with 3 in each group.
4. One group along with two unvaccinated guinea pigs serving as control are challenged with *Clostridium septicum* and other group along with two controls with *Clostridium chauvei.*
5. All the controls should die within 3-5 days with no death in vaccinated animals, confirms potency of the manufactured vaccine.

The shelf life of the vaccine is two years provided stored at 4°C. The vaccine is recommended against Black-quarter and malignant oedema infections in cattle and sheep at the dose rate of 5ml and 3ml S/C respectively.

H.S. Alum Precipitated Vaccine

Seed Culture

The organism *Pasturella multocida* strain 52 is procured from IVRI, Izatnagar and maintained in the laboratory with animal passages in calf. The calf is inoculated with the broth culture and soon after the death or just before the death of animal, heart blood is collected in sterilized vials and sealed while observing strict asepsis. The blood so collected may be incubated for overnight to concentrate the organisms and then stored in refrigerator or kept as such in a dark cool place. Small quantity of this blood is aspirated from the vials and streaked out on blood agar plates and incubated overnight. The individual colonies are examined for pasturella and single colony is transferred into nutrient broth and incubated overnight. The growth in broth is examined and growth, if pure and sufficient, serves as primary culture. The seed is maintained by inoculating the blood from vials every 6 monthly in a natural susceptible host.

Culture Medium

The medium required to culture the pasturella -52 contains;

1. Peptone-1%
2. Beef extract-1.5%
3. Yeast extract-1%
4. Sodium chloride-0.5%, and
5. pH is adjusted to 7.4 with sodium hydroxide.

Procedure

1. Prepare the medium, dispense it in solution bottles of 5 or 10 litres.
2. Autoclave it at 15lb pressure for 45 minutes.
3. The autoclaved medium is tested for sterility by incubating it overnight.
4. Select the bottles with sterile medium for vaccine production.
5. Inoculate the selected bottles with primary seed culture at 50ml per bottle in laminar flow.
6. Seal the bottles and incubate at 37°C for 24 hours.
7. Examine the growth for its purity by staining technique. Any undesired growth in the medium makes it liable to be discarded.
8. Formalization of pure growth is done by adding formalin at concentration of 0.5% in the product i.e. 5ml per litre of culture broth and mix it well.
9. The product is tested for sterility after 24 hours of formalization by incubating it in a fresh medium.
10. Before bottling, autoclaved alum is added at a concentration of 1% in the product and blended with the help of electric churner.
11. Bottling, sealing and labeling of alum precipitated product is carried out as per the laboratory standards.

The shelf life of the vaccine is 6 months when stored at refrigeration temperature and dose in large animals is 5ml S/c.

Quality Control Tests

Sterility Test

1. 3% of samples from the vaccine batch are taken randomly.
2. Inoculation of samples into fresh aerobic as well as anaerobic broth tubes is carried out.
3. Inoculated tubes are incubated for 48-72 hours.
4. No growth confirms its being sterile.

Safety and Potency Tests

1. 4 albino white mice are inoculated, two with 0.5ml and two with 1ml intraperitoneally.

2. They are observed for 5 days and no death labels the vaccine as safe.
3. For potency test three calves are inoculated with 3ml of vaccine S/C and observed for any untoward reaction for a week.
4. The vaccinated calves along with two unvaccinated calves, serving as control, are challenged with 1ml of 18 hours old broth culture of pasturella.
5. Both the control animals should die and all vaccinated animals should survive which indicates the success of vaccination.
6. Safe and potent vaccine is ready to be used in field.

H.S Oil Adjuvant Vaccine

Seed Culture

The seed used and maintained is the same as in H.S. alum precipitated vaccine. (See above)

Culture Medium

In oil adjuvant vaccine growth is obtained from solid medium which in this case contains;

1. Peptone-1%
2. Yeast extract-0.5%
3. Sodium chloride-0.5%
4. Agar powder-3-4%, and
5. pH is adjusted to 7.4.

Procedure

1. Prepared medium is dispensed in roux flasks at 150ml per flask.
2. Plugging and sealing with non-absorbent cotton and tin foil is done.
3. Medium is sterilized by autoclaving at 15lbs pressure for 45 minutes.
4. After autoclaving, the flasks are placed horizontally and allowed to cool to form a uniform layer of medium.

5. The flasks are tested for sterility by incubating them overnight and only sterile flasks are selected for production of vaccine.
6. 3 to 5ml of primary seed culture is inoculated in each of the selected flasks and spread over the medium by to and fro movement of the flask.
7. Incubation of the inoculated flasks is carried at 37°C for 24 hours.
8. Growth is washed using 0.5%formal saline 10-15ml per flask and sterilized glass beads.
9. Flasks are washed two to three times to ensure complete washing of the growth.
10. The growth is examined for purity from each of the flask by staining technique.
11. Washings from the flasks with desirable growth are pooled together.
12. The opacity of the washing is to be adjusted between tube 6 and 7 (standardized tubes) by diluting it with 0.5% formalin-saline.
13. The product is tested for sterility by inoculating in a fresh medium.
14. 15 parts of washed bacterial suspension is mixed with 10 parts of sterilized liquid paraffin and 1 part of lanolin.
15. The mixture is blended in an electric churner till a white creamy, uniform and stable emulsion is produced.
16. Bottling, sealing and labeling of the final product is done as per the laboratory standards.

The shelf-life of the vaccine is about a year when stored at refrigeration temperature. The adult dose is 3ml intramuscularly.

Quality Control Tests

Safety and Sterility

1. The vaccine thus prepared is subjected to sterility tests by inoculating it in a fresh aerobic as well as anaerobic culture tubes
2. Incubation is carried out for 24-72 hours.
3. No growth in the medium certifies it sterile.

4. The vaccine is injected intraperitoneally in white albino mice at 0.5ml and observed for 5 days.
5. No death from pasturellosis, renders vaccine safe for use.

Potency Test

1. Inject intramuscularly 2-3 ml of finished product in calves.
2. Observe the animals for any rise in temperature or reaction up to a week.
3. Challenge the vaccinated calves with 1ml of 18 hours old broth culture of pasturella along with two unvaccinated calves serving as control.
4. Both the control animals should die and all vaccinated animals should survive which indicates successful vaccination.
5. Safe and potent vaccine is ready to be used in field.

Combined Oil Adjuvant H.S and B.Q Vaccine

The two vaccines, H.S and B.Q are prepared as formalized broths as described above. One part of H.S formalized broth and 2-3 parts of B.Q formalized broth are centrifuged together at 3000rpm at refrigeration. Twelve parts of sediment are mixed with ten parts of liquid paraffin and two parts of lanolin to which is added Tween 80-2%. This procedure is simple but requires commercial refrigeration centrifuges.

Ranikhet Disease Vaccine

Seed Culture

The seed is procured from IVRI, Izatnagar in a freeze dried condition. The seed is tested for its ED-50 by serially diluting the seed with normal saline and inoculated in embryonated eggs. The embryonic deaths are recorded in different dilutions and the dilution at which there is only 50% embryonic mortality is referred as ED50.

Culture medium

Live embryonated eggs.

Procedure

1. Specific pathogen free, ten days (for R_2B) or nine days (for F_1) live, vigorously moving embryonated eggs are procured from the hatchery.

2. The egg shells are disinfected with tincture iodine or 70% alcohol.
3. Air sacs are chalked out while candling the eggs, with a marker pencil.
4. The inoculation site, which is allantoic route (see chapter 6), is chalked out. While selecting the inoculation site, care is taken to avoid blood vessels.
5. Inoculation is employed either by making a single puncture just 2-3mm above air sac line and needle is pierced vertically via sac in to the allantoic space or by drilling one puncture in the center of air sac and other puncture just below the air sac line avoiding vascular net work and needle is pierced horizontally in to the allantoic sac.
6. The seed is diluted with normal saline to ED-50 and inoculation is carried out in 10 days (for R_2B vaccine production) or 9 days (for F_1 vaccine production) live, embryonated eggs.
7. In all the cases the puncture sites are sealed with paraffin wax or cellophane tape or nail polish.
8. The inoculated eggs are incubated at 38°C in egg incubator for 40-60 hours in R_2B and 70-96 hours in F_1 strains
9. Candling is made after 24 hours and eggs with dead embryos discarded. This should not, however, be above 5% which otherwise indicates wrong inoculation or infection or incubation failure.
10. After required incubation with more than 50% embryos dead, the eggs are taken out from the incubator.
11. Eggs are then placed in the refrigerator for few hours before collection of fluid, to ensure the death of embryos and collapsing of blood vessels so that during collection, blood does not get mixed with the collection fluid.
12. The egg shell is cut along the air sac line.
13. Egg shell membrane is peeled off with the help of toothed forceps.
14. The chorioallantoic membranes are ruptured and fluid is collected with the help of automatic pipette or a pipette attached to a suction pump.

15. The fluid thus obtained is collected into vials or flasks on ice. 2-5ml of fluid gets collected from each egg.
16. All these procedures of egg inoculation or fluid collection are carried out in a laminar flow while observing strict aseptic measures.
17. The fluid collected from each egg is subjected to spot HA test and fluids with satisfactory HA are pooled together.
18. Antibiotics like streptomycin 100mg and penicillin 100iu per ml of fluid are added, besides skimmed milk at concentration of 5% in the fluid.
19. The fluid is mixed properly in a mixer.
20. H.A titre is evaluated in the pooled collection and fluid with satisfactory virus content is then dispensed in the cryo-resistant vials in the amounts of 1ml or 2ml.
21. The vials are stored at -20°C before loading into lyophilizer.
22. Lyophilization of the vaccine is carried out in preset electronically monitored lyophilizer.

The shelf-life of the vaccine is one year when stored at -20°C. Dose of RD(R_2B) vaccine is 0.5ml S/C at the age of 6-8 weeks and for F_1 vaccine one drop intranasal at the age of 5-9 days. The vaccine is reconstituted in normal saline and reconstituted vaccine should be used within 2 hours.

Quality Control Tests

Sterility and Safety Tests

1. The vaccine is inoculated in aerobic as well as anaerobic culture media and incubated for 24-72 hours.
2. Any growth in the medium renders the vaccine unsafe for the field use.
3. R_2B vaccine is injected in 3 healthy chickens subcutaneously with 0.1ml of vaccine having strength ten times more than the usual dose of the vaccine.
4. F_1 vaccine is given in 5 healthy, day old chicks, two drops intranasal.
5. The birds are observed for two weeks for any septicemia or infection. The safe vaccine is then subjected to potency tests.

Potency Tests

1. Birds of 8-12 weeks age are vaccinated with the R_2B test vaccine where as chicks from day one to nine days are vaccinated with test F_1 vaccine.
2. In R_2B vaccine, two weeks after the vaccination, the birds are challenged with 0.5ml of 1:100 dilution of virulent virus (liver or spleen suspension or fluid from infected embryo) along with two unvaccinated birds serving as control.
3. In F1 vaccine, 14 days after vaccination, the chicks are challenged with 2drops, intranasal, of 1:50 dilution of virulent RD virus along with 4 unprotected chicks.
4. The control birds in both test vaccinations should develop symptoms of RKD and die where as none from the vaccinated group should die during observation period of 14 days. This labels the vaccine potent.
5. Safe and potent vaccine should be used in the field.

Table 8.1: Vaccination Schedule for Livestock and Poultry.

Species	*Diseases*	*Vaccine Brands & Dose*	*Vaccination Schedule*
Cattle	FMD	(a) Hoescht FMD vaccine (trivalent) *@ 5ml S/C.* (b) Raksha Ovac (trivalent oil adjuvant). *@ 3ml S/C.* (c) Baif FMD vaccine (trivalent) *@ 3ml S/C.*	*Enzootic areas*: 3-4 times a year, starting from one month of age. *Sporadic areas*: twice a year, starting from 3-4 months of age. *Pregnant animals* to be avoided during early and late pregnancy.
Cattle	RP	(a) GTV RP vaccine *@ 5ml S/C or I/M* (b) Chick embryo RP vaccine *@ 5ml S/C or I/M.*	Annual vaccination (conducted only in endemic areas, border villages, ring vaccination and selected herd vaccination). However, RP vaccination in India has been stopped from 2001 and only sero-surveillance is being carried out presently by Government of India.
Cattle	IBR	IBRIVAX (BHV-1), oil adjuvant vaccine *@ 2ml S/C*	Annual vaccination. In Kashmir valley sero-prevalence of IBR has been reported as high as 35-50% in different areas.
Cattle	H.S & B.Q	(a) H.S or B.Q formalized broth vaccine *@ 5ml S/C.* (b) H.S oil adjuvant *@ 3ml I/M* (c) Raksha Biovac (FMD + HS oil adjuvant). *@ 5ml S/C.* (d) Raksha Triovac(FMD + HS + BQ oil adjuvant). *@ 5ml S/C.*	Twice or once a year.

contd...

Table 8.1–Contd...

Species	*Diseases*	*Vaccine Brands & Dose*	*Vaccination Schedule*
Cattle, Sheep, Goat, Dog	Rabies	Embryo adapted or cell inactivated vaccines like Nobivac, Rakshrab, Rabisin or Rabipur @ *1ml S/C or I.M*	*Post bite:* 0 day, 3rd day, 7th day, 14th day, 22nd day and booster on 90th day. *Prophylactic*: 8-12 weeks age in dogs, small ruminants and horse. Revaccination annually.
Cattle, Sheep, Goats, Foals	Tetanus	Alum precipitated formalized vaccines (a) Anti-tetanus toxoid (ATT) (b) Tetanus toxoid (TT) @ *1ml -2ml I/M* (c) TIG –Tetanus immuno-globulin (hyper immune serum) at *time of risk.*	Repeat the injection after one month and booster after 8-10 months confers protection up to 8 years.
Sheep	Entero-toxaemia Eraxy	(a) MCCV- Multicomponant clostredial vaccine *@ 5ml I/P.* (b) Alum precipitated toxoid *@ 2ml S/C.*	Two doses at 2 weeks apart and annual revaccination.
Horse	African Horse Sickness	(a) AHS vaccine (polyvalent tissue inactivated) (b) Formalin killed alum precipitated vaccine.	Two doses one month apart. Protection for 6 months in enzootic areas.
Poultry	RKD	(a) *RD F_1 vaccine @ 1drop intranasal or intra ocular.* (b) *RD R_2B vaccine @ 0.5ml S/C or I/M.* (c) *RD lasota vaccine @ 1000 doses in 15 litres of drinking water for 5-6 weeks olo and in 25 litres for 15-16 weeks old bids.*	F_1 at 5 – 9 days age. R_2B at 6 weeks age if needed revaccination can be done after 8-10 months preferably 14 days after giving F vaccine. Lasota vaccine is given in 5-6 week old or 15-16 week old layers. May be repeated every 3 months.

contd...

Table 8.1–Contd...

Species	*Diseases*	*Vaccine Brands & Dose*	*Vaccination Schedule*
Poultry	Spiro-chaetosis	Freeze dried vaccine *@ 1ml I/M*	Vaccination above 6 weeks of age.
Poultry	IBD	IBD vaccine *@ 1000 doses in 8 litres of drinking water with 50g skimmed milk.*	Vaccination in 18-21 days old chicks. May be repeated at 7th week of age.
Poultry	Marek's disease	Freeze dried turkey herpes virus *@ 0.2ml S/C or I/M*	Vaccination in day old chicks may be repeated annually.
Poultry	IB	Avian infectious bronchitis vaccine. *@ 1 drop intranasal or in drinking water as in Lasota.*	Nasal drop vaccination in 5-10 days old chicks and booster in drinking water at 6-8 weeks age which may be repeated at 14-16 weeks age.

Chapter 9

Physiological Profile of Various Parameters in Different Animals

Table 9.1: Normal Haematological Profile In Different Animals.

Parameter	*Cattle*	*Sheep*	*Goat*	*Pig*	*Horse*	*Dog*	*Cat*	*Fowl*	*Man*
Hb (g%)	8-14 (11)	8-16 (12)	8-14 (11)	11-17 (14)	8-14 (11)	12-18 (15)	8-14 (12)	7-11	13-15
PCV (%)	24-38 (32)	26-36 (30)	24-36 (30)	37-50 (42)	24-44 (35)	37-55 (45)	24-45 (37)	27- 42	41-52
RBC (10^6/cumm)	5-9 (7)	5-11 (8)	10-18 (13)	6-9 (7.2)	5.5- 9.5 (7.5)	5.5-8.5 (6.4)	5.5-10 (7.5)	2.5- 3.2	4 -6
Diameter of RBC (μ)	5.9	4.8	4	6	5.5	7	6	11.2x 6.8	7.5
RBC Surface Area (sq.μ)	110	66	50	113	84	121	113	183	162

Contd...

Table 9.1–Contd...

Parameter	*Cattle*	*Sheep*	*Goat*	*Pig*	*Horse*	*Dog*	*Cat*	*Fowl*	*Man*
RBC Surface Area (sq.m/ kg b.wt.)	62	58	56	63	67	68	63	44	65
Total RBC Surface Area (sq. m)	30800	2323	1680	6328	33600	1355	190	88	4536
MCV (cu μ)	46-54	35	19	58	42	59-69	51-63	115-125	82-96
MCH (pg)	15-20	13	7	19	3	20-24	13-17	25-27	29-32
MCHC (%)	32-39	35	35	33	33	30-35	32-34	21-23	30-36
WBC (10^3/cumm)	4 -10 (7)	4 -10 (8)	4 -13 (8)	10-23 (18)	6-12 (8)	6-15 (10)	7-20 (12.5)	20-33	5 -10
Neutrophils (%)	15-45 (28)	10-50 (30)	30-40 (36)	28-47 (37)	35-75 (55)	55-75 (62)	35-75 (59)	25-30	55-70
Lympho-cytes (%)	55-75 (58)	50-75 (62)	50-70 (56)	40-65 (59)	15-50 (35)	15-30 25)	20-55 (32)	50-59	25-70
Monocytes (%)	2-7 (4)	0-6 (2.5)	0-4 (2.5)	2-10 (5)	2-10 (5)	3-10 (5.5)	1-4 (3)	7-10	3-7
Eosinophils (%)	0-20 (9)	0-10 (5)	1-8 (5)	1-11 (3.5)	2-12 (5)	2-10 (7)	2-12 (5.5)	3 -8	1-4
Basophils (%)	0-2 (0.5)	0-3 (0.5)	0-1 (0.5)	0-2 (0.5)	0-3 (0.5)	00	00	0 -2	0-1
Platelets (10^6/cumm)	0.2-0.6	0.25-0.75	0.2-0.5	0.25-0.70	0.2-0.6	0.2-0.5	0.3-0.6	0.02-0.04	0.35- 0.45
ESR (mm)	2-6/ 24 hrs	00/hr.	00/hr.	1-14/hr.	50/hr.	6-10/hr.	7-27/hr.	1-3/hr.	8-10/hr.
Heart Rate (beats/min)	60-70	70-80	70-80	55-86	32-44	90-120	110-140	200-400	60-90

Contd...

Table 9.1–Contd...

Parameter	*Cattle*	*Sheep*	*Goat*	*Pig*	*Horse*	*Dog*	*Cat*	*Fowl*	*Man*
Blood Volume (ml/kg)	59-85	58-74	70	58-95	68	92	70	40-50	70
Plasma Volume (ml/kg)	37-54	46-53	53	36-50	43-63	43-58	46-48	46	50
Mean Blood Pressure (mm Hg)	125-166	110	120	169	169	150	140-170	135	100
Cardiac Output (ml/kg/min)	99-113	107 -114	129		75	138	69	121-171	70
Bleeding Time (min)	5.5	1-4	1-4	1-4		1-4	1-4	1-4	2-6
Clotting Time (min)	6.5	1.5 – 2.5	2.5	3.5	11.5	2.5	1.5	4.5	4 -10
Rectal Temp.(°F)	101.5	102.3	103.8	102.5	99.7	102	101.5	107	98.4
Respiration Rate(breaths /min)	30	19	19	16	12	22	26	15-30	12-20
Passive (*prenatal*)	00	00	00	00	00	+	+	++	+++
Immunity Transmission (*postnatal*)	+++ 24 hr	+++ 24 hr	+++ 24 hr	+++ 24-36 hr	+++ 24 hr	++ 1-2 day	++ 1-2 day	++ <5day	00

Table 9.2: Values of Chemical Constituents of Blood In Different Animals.

Parameter	*Cattle*	*Sheep*	*Goat*	*Pig*	*Horse*	*Dog*	*Cat*	*Fowl*	*Man*
Blood Glucose (mg%)	35-55	35-74	45-60	80-120	55-95	70-100	80-120	130-260	70-100
Blood NPN (mg%)	20-40	20-38	30-44	20-45	20-40	17-38	-	20-36	25-40
Blood Urea Nitrogen (mg%)	6-27	8-20	13-28	8-24	10-20	10-20	20-30	0.4 -1	9-12
Blood Uric Acid (mg%)	0.05-2	0.05-2	0.3-1	0.05-2	0.9-1	0-0.5	-	1-2	2-4.5
Blood Creatinine (mg%)	1-2	1-2	1-2	1-2	1-2	1-2	1-2	1-2	1-2
Blood Aminoacid Nitrogen (mg%)	4 -8	5-8	-	8	5-7	7-8	-	5-10	-
Blood Lactic Acid (mg%)	5-20	9-12	-	-	10-16	8-20	-	47-98	-
Total Plasma Protein (g%)	6.74 –7.46	6.00- 7.90	6.40- 7.90	7.9 – 8.9	5.70 – 7.80	5.40 – 7.10	5.40 – 7.30	5.6	7.5
Albumin (g%)	3.03 -3.55	2.70 -3.90	2.70 -3.90	1.80 – 3.30	2.33 – 3.85	2.30 -3.20	2.10 -3.30	2.5	-
Globulin (g%)	3.00 – 3.48	3.50 -5.70	2.70 -4.10	5.29 – 6.43	2.62 -4.04	2.70 -4.40	2.60 -5.10	3.1	-
Fibrinogen (mg%)	450-700	-	-	-	200-400	200-400	200-400	-	200-400
Serum Total Cholesterol (mg%)	50-230	100-150	55-200	100-250	75-150	125-250	90-110	58-94	150-250

Contd...

Table 9.2–Contd...

Parameter	*Cattle*	*Sheep*	*Goat*	*Pig*	*Horse*	*Dog*	*Cat*	*Fowl*	*Man*
Total Triglycerides (mg%)	0-14				4 -44				
Serum Calcium (mg%)	9.4-12.2	11.4	10.7	11	12-13.4	9.8-11.6	8.22	9-12	9-11
Serum Phosphorus (mg%)	4 -7.12	5.1-9	3-11	4 -11	2.4 -4.2	2.2-4	6.4	4 -8	2-4
Serum Magnesium (mg%)	2-5	2-5	2-3	2-3	2.5	2.1	2-3	5-9	2-4
Sodium(mEq/L)	142	153	-	155	149	143	151	-	-
Potassium(mEq/L)	4.8	4.8	-	5.9	3.3	4.4	4.3	-	-
Chloride (mEq/L)	104	116	-	103	102	106	120	-	-
Bicarbonate (mEq/L)	21.5	20.5	-	-	23.0	18.6	18	-	-
pH	7.35-7.50	7.44	-	-	7.20-7.55	7.36	7.35	-	-
Phosphate (mg%)	5.6-6.5	6.9	-	5.3-9.6	3.1-5.6	5.6	-	7.81	-
Bilirubin (mg%)	0.01-0.47	0-0.39	0 - 0.1	0 – 0.6	0.2 – 2.0	0.07 – 0.61	0.15 – 0.20	-	-
Alkaline Phosphatase (iu/L)	0 - 38	5 – 30	7 - 30	9 - 31	11 - 31	3 -16	2 - 7	-	-
Lactate Dehydrogenase (LDH) (iu/L)	176-365	60-111	31-99	96-160	41-104	10-35	16-69	636	-
SGOT (iu/L)	20-34	68-80	43-132	8.2-21.6	58-94	6-18	6.7-11	-	-
SGPT (iu/L)	4 -11	10-12	7-24	9 -17	1 – 6.7	4.8 - 24	1.7 - 14	-	-
Serum Thyroxine (ug%)	4.10±0.7	3.70±0.6	5.25±2.08	3.50±0.5	1.47±0.21	1.10±0.59	0.95±0.5		

Table: 9.3: Cerebrospinal Fluid Chemistry In Different Animals.

Substances	*Cattle*	*Sheep*	*Goat*	*Pig*	*Horse*	*Dog*	*Cat*	*Fowl*	*Man*
pH	7.2	7.3-7.4	-	-	7.1-7.3	7.1-7.3	7.2	-	-
WBC Cells per µl	0-6	0-5	0-4	0-7	1-7	0-25	0-1	-	-
Pressure (mmwater)	<200	60-270		80-145	272-490	24-172	100	-	-
Rate of Formation (µl/m)	290	118	164			47-66	20-22	-	-
Total protein (mg%)	23.4-66.3	29-42	12	24-29	40-170	18-44	0-30	-	-
Albumin (mg%)	8.2-28.7	-	-	17-24	22.6-67.9	7.5-27.6	19-25	-	-
Globulin (mg%)	-	-	-	5-10	3.4-18.4	14-21	-	-	-
Calcium (mg%)	5.1-6.3	5.1-5.5	4.6		2.5-6.0	5.1-7.4	5.1-6.3	-	-
Phosphorus (mg%)	0.9-2.5	1.2-2	-	-	0.5-1.5	2.8-3.4	-	-	-
Sodium (mmol/L)	132-142	145-157	131	134-144	140-150	151-155	158	-	-
Potassium (mmol/L)	2.7-3.2	3-3.3	3	-	2.5-3.5	2.9-3.2	-	-	-
Urea nitrogen (mg%)	8-11	-	-	-	0-20	4.7-5.1	10-11	-	-
Glucose (mg%)	37-51	52-85	70	45-87	30-70	48-57	18-130	-	-

Table 9.4: Physiological Values Of Reproductive Cycles In Different Females.

Parameter	*Cow*	*Ewe*	*Doe (Goat)*	*Sow*	*Mare*	*Bitch*	*Cat*
Length of Estrous (days)	21	17	20	21	21	Estrous at 4 -8 month interval	Seasonal polyestrous - Spring &fall
Length of Estrous	18 hr.	29 hr.	40 hr.	45 hr.	5 days	7-9 days	4 days
Time of Ovulation	11 hr after end of estrous	Near end of estrous	33 hr after start of estrous	24-36 hr after start of estrous	3rd -6th day of estrous	2nd-3rd day of estrous	27 hr post - coitus
Fertilized Ova Enter Uterus (days)	4, post-estrous	4, post-estrous	4, post-estrous	3-4, post coitus	-	5-6, post-coitus	4, after ovulation
Implantation Begins at (days)	35, post estrous	15, post estrous	20, post estrous	10, post estrous	56, post estrous	15, post coitus	13, post coitus
Length of Pregnancy (days)	282	148	148	115	335	63	63
Type of Placenta	Epithelio-chorial	Syndes-mochorial	Syndes-mochorial	Epithelio-chorial	Epithelio-chorial	Endothe-liochorial	Endothe-liochorial
Puberty Age (Months)	10-14	6-12	6-12	6-12	10-18	7-12	-

Table 9.5: Measurements Of Gastrointestinal Tract In Different Animals. (Relative Capacity %)

Parameter	*Cattle*	*Sheep*	*Goat*	*Pig*	*Horse*	*Dog*	*Cat*
Stomach	71	67	67	29	9	63	69
Small Intestine	18	21	21	33	30	23	15
Caecum	3	2	2	6	16	1	-
Colon & Rectum	8	10	10	32	45	13	16
		%age of Weight of Whole Stomach					
Rumen and Reticulum	64	69	69				
Omasum	25	8	8				
Abomasums	11	23	23				

Table 9.6: Cranial Nerves.

Number	*Name*	*Function*	*Location*
I	Olfactory	Sensory	Anterior of brain
II	Optic	Sensory	Anterior to pituitary
III	Oculomotor	Motor	Posterior to pituitary
IV	Trochlear	Motor	Posterior to colliculi
V	Trigeminal	Mixed	Ventral pons
VI	Abducent	Motor	Posteroventral pons
VII	Facial	Mixed	Posteroventral pons
VIII	Acoustic	Sensory	Posteroventral pons
IX	Glossopharyngeal	Mixed	Lateral medulla
X	Vagus	Mixed	Lateral medulla
XI	Spinal accessory	Motor	Lateral medulla
XII	hypoglossal	Motor	Lateral medulla

Table 9.7: Physiological Values Of Semen In Different Animals.

Semen Parameters	*Bull*	*Horse*	*Ram*	*Pig*	*Dog*	*Cat*	*Fowl*
Volume (ml)	4	70	1	250	10	0.04	0.5
Sperm Conc. (million/ml)	1200	120	3000	150	125	1730	4000
Sperm Head (μ) Length/width	9.15/4.25	5/2.4	8.2/4.25	8.5/4.25	7/4		
Middle Piece (μ) Length/width	14.84/0.67	8/0.50	14/0.80	10/-	10	-	-
Tail Piece (μ) Length/width	45-50/0.51	30/0.49	40-45/0.50	30/-	34	-	-
pH	6.8	7.4	6.8	7.5	6.7	7.4	7.02-7.18
Sodium (mg%)	230	70	190	650	90	-	-
Potassium (mg%)	140	60	90	240	8:2	-	-
Calcium (mg%)	44	20	10	5	0.7	-	-
Magnesium (mg%)	9	3	8	11	0.5	-	
Chloride (mg%)	180	270	86	330	630	-	-
Phosphorus (Total mg)	82	19	357	142	13	-	-
Fructose (mg%)	530	2	250	13	trace	-	-
Glycerylphos-phoryl Choline (mg%)	350	80	1650	180	180	-	-
Citric Acid (mg%)	700	25	140	80	trace	-	-
Lactic Acid (mg%)	30	15	40	30	-	-	-
Ascorbic Acid (mg%)	6	-	5	-	-	-	-
Inositol (mg%)	35	30	12	530	-	-	-
Sorbitol (mg%)	10-140	40	92	12	0	-	-
Ergothioneine	trace	7.6	trace	15	-	-	-
Spermine	0	0	0	0	0	-	-

Table 9.8: Composition of Milk in Different Animals.

Species	*Fat (%)*	*Protein (%)*	*Lactose (%)*	*Ash (%)*
Buffalo	7.7	4.3	4.7	0.8
Bitch	9.5	9.3	3.1	1.2
Cattle (holstein)	3.5	3.1	4.9	0.7
Cattle (jersey)	5.5	3.9	4.9	0.7
Cattle (zebu)	4.9	3.9	5.1	0.8
Goat	3.5	3.1	4.6	0.8
Human	4.3	1.4	6.9	0.2
Mare	1.6	2.4	6.1	0.5
Sheep	10.4	6.8	3.7	0.9
Swine	7.9	5.9	4.9	0.9
Yak	7.0	5.2	4.6	—

Table 9.9: Composition of Egg.

Composition	*Yolk*	*Outer Thin*	*Middle Thick*	*Inner Thin*	*Chalazi-ferous*	*Shell*
Weight(g)	18.7	7.6	18.9	5.5	0.9	6.2
Water (%)	48.7	88.8	87.6	86.4	84.3	1.6
Solids (%)	51.3	11.2	12.4	13.6	15.7	98.4
Protein (%)	16.6		10.60			3.3
Carbohydrate (%)	1		0.9			—
Fats (%)	32.6		Traces			0.03
Minerals (%)	1.1		0.6			95.1

Table 9.10: Urine Analyte in Different Animals.

Parameters	*Cattle*	*Sheep*	*Goat*	*Pig*	*Horse*	*Dog*	*Cat*	*Man*
Volume of Urine (ml/kg /day)	17-45	10-40	10-40	5-30	3-18	17-45	10-20	9-28
Specific Gravity of Urine	1.032	1.030	1.030	1.012	1.040	1.025	1.030	1.020
pH	7.4-8.4	7.4-8.4	7.4-8.4	5-8	7-8	5-7	5-7	—
Total Nitrogen (mg/kg/day)	40-450	120-350	120-400	40-240	100-600	250-800	500-1100	—
Uric acid (mg/kg/day)	1-4	2-4	2-5	1-2	1-2	—	—	—

Table 9.11: Physiological Data of Different Laboratory Animals.

Data	*Rabbits*	*Guinea Pigs*	*Mice*	*Rat*	*Hamster*
Rectal Temperature(°F)	101.6-102.4	99.6- 102	99.3	99.5	98-101
Normal Respiration Rate /min	55	80	—	210	—
Pulse Rate /min.	135	150	120	—	—
Gestation Period (days)	28-31	63	19-21	21-23	16-17
Weaning Age (weeks)	6-8	2-3	3	3-4	3-4
Mating Age (weeks)	30-36	12-20	6-8	10-12	7-9
Litters(per year)	4	3	8-12	7-9	3-4
Litter Size	4	3	7-8	7	6
Room Temperature(°F)	60-65	65-70	68-70	65-70	68-72
Humidity (%)	40-45	45	50-60	45-55	40-50
Eyes Open (Days After Birth)	10	Prior to birth	11-14	14-17	15
Breeding Life (Years)	1-3	3-4	1-1½	1	1- 1½
Life Span (Years)	5-7	4-5	3-3½	3	2-3
Weight (Adult) (gm)	0.9 – 6075	200-1000	25-28	—	—

Addresses of Different Diagnostic Laboratories in India

1. Center for Animal Disease Research and Diagnosis (CADRAD), Indian Veterinary Institute, Izatnagar, U.P.
2. National Institute of Virology, 20-A, Dr. Ambadkhar Road, Pune-411001.
3. Royal Western India Turf Club (RWITC) Laboratory, Pune, Maharashtra.
4. Project Coordinator, All India Coordinated Research Project (AICRP) for Epidemiological Studies, Mukteswar, Kumaon, Nanital- 263138.
5. High Security Animal Disease Laboratory, Halthai Kedhar Road, Anand Nagar, Bhopal-46202 M.P.
6. Industrial Toxicology Research Center, Mahatma Gandhi Marg, Lucknow -226001, U.P.
7. Regional Disease Diagnostic Laboratory, Ludhiana, Punjab.
8. Project Directorate on Animal Disease Monitoring and Surveillance, Hebbal, Bangalore.
9. Directorate of Forensic Science Laboratory, Srinagar, J & K.

Index

S

T

U

V

W

X

Y

Z